Alkaline Diet & Anti-Inflammatory Diet For Beginners:

The Ultimate Guide To Eat Healty, Fight Inflammation, Lose Weight and Fight Chronic Disease

James Fitt

Table of Contents

INTRODUCTION

When you choose to eat an alkaline diet, you are actually eating foods that are very similar to what man was designed to eat. If you look at what our ancestors ate, you will find a diet rich in fresh fruits, vegetables, legumes, nuts, and fish. Unfortunately, man's diet today is frequently full of foods that are high in unhealthy fats, salt, cholesterol, and acidifying foods.

How Our Diet Changed

Although some people think that man's diet changed only recently, the shift from a largely alkaline diet to an acid diet actually began thousands of years ago. Our original diet consisted of foraged fruits, nuts and vegetables, along with whatever meat could be caught. As soon as man started to grow his own food, things started to change. Grains became a popular diet choice, especially after the development of stone tools. Once animals were domesticated, there were dairy products added to the diet, along with an additional amount of meat. Salt began to be added, along with sugar. The end result was a diet that was still much healthier than what many people eat today, but the shift from alkaline to acid had begun.

Recent Dietary Changes

It's no secret that our modern diet consists of many foods which are not healthy for us. Too much junk food and "fast food" has decreased the quality of our diet. Obesity has become the norm, and along with it a higher incidence of diseases such as diabetes, coronary disease, and cancer. If you want to improve your health and reduce the risk of many diseases, an alkaline diet can help get your body back to basics.

What is an Alkaline Diet?

When foods are eaten and digested, they produce either an acidifying or alkalizing effect within the body. Some people get confused because the actual pH of the food itself doesn't have anything to do with the

effect of the food once it is digested. When more alkaline foods are consumed, the body can become slightly alkaline instead of acid. Ideally, the blood pH level should be between 7.35 and 7.45. Foods such as citrus fruits, soy products, raw fruits and vegetables, wild rice, almonds, and natural sweeteners such as Stevia are all good alkaline food choices.

Benefits of an Alkaline Diet

There are many benefits to shifting your eating patterns from acid to alkaline. When the body is kept slightly alkaline, it is less susceptible to disease. It's easier to lose weight or maintain a healthy weight level on an alkaline diet. Most people experience an increase in their energy level, as well as a lessening of anxiety and irritability once they begin eating more alkaline foods. Mucous production is decreased and nasal congestion is reduced, making it easier to breath. Allergies are frequently alleviated as a result of an alkaline diet. The body is also less susceptible to illnesses such as cancer and diabetes. Most people find that they just feel better, with an increased sense of health and well- being, once they make a conscious effort to adhere to an alkaline diet.

WHAT IS ALKALINE DIET

There are many alkaline diet guidelines. The basic idea is certain substances are worse for the body then others. One of the alkaline diet guidelines is that you should attempt to eat 75-80% alkaline. Meaning that 75-80% of your diet is from the alkaline food chart. Certain foods are considered more acid forming than others though. To give you an idea here is a list of foods that are considered highly acid forming according to the alkaline diet guidelines: sweeteners (equal, sweet and low, nutra-sweet, and aspartame to name a few) beer, table salt, jam, ice cream, beef, lobster, fried food, processed cheese, and soft drinks. Here is a fun fact cola has ph of 2.5. This is highly acidic. In order to neutralize on can of cola you would have to drink 32 glasses of water.

On the other side of the spectrum, there are certain food that are considered to by highly alkaline and when ingested help increase the alkalinity of the body. According to the alkaline diet guidelines, these food are as follows: sea salt, lotus rood, watermelon, tangerines, sweet potato, lime, pineapple, seaweed, pumpkin seeds, and lentils.

The alkaline diet guidelines say that drugs are extremely acid forming as well. Think about all those people who take some form of drug to ease their acid reflux. Little do they know their temporary solution is causing bigger problems for them in the long run. There are many other alkaline diet foods this was just an example. The more you eat the better you will feel. Many times people experience a period of detoxification when they switch to the alkaline diet. The alkaline diet guidelines suggest that you got through a period of a couple of weeks in detox to rid your body of toxins and allow to adjust to this completely new way of eating.

WHAT IS AN ACID ALKALINE DIET

A lot of people have been struggling to find the best diet program fit for them. One of the most common misrepresentation that these people have is their desire to lose weight. They fail to put vital emphasis on how to be healthy. If you want to know the best diet that is perfect for you, then you better make sure it's healthy and is not destroying your body.

The Alkaline Diet

Surely, you have encountered an alkaline meal program somewhere online or in some reading materials. What is an alkaline diet and is this diet healthy for you? This diet all started when experts tried considering the pH level of the body. In a person's body, the environment can be acidic or alkaline. Once the pH level is high then the environment is alkaline. In contrary, low pH means the environment is acidic. The body does not have one single pH level rather it can differ depending on the location. The pH level in the stomach is different from the urinary bladder.

This diet is basically all about eating foods which can promote alkaline environment in the body while not eating foods that promote acidity to the body. What could be the reason behind this program? To start off, foods that can promote an alkaline environment in the body, are considered healthy. Examples of these foods include vegetables, fruits, soy products, nuts, legumes, and cereals. If you have noticed, these foods are rich in protein, vitamins, and minerals.

Th other principle of an alkaline diet is to avoid acid foods because these are foods that can make your body at risk for weight gain, heart problems, kidney and liver diseases. Few of the many acid foods include caffeine, foods with high preservatives like canned goods, sodas, fish, meat, alcohol and foods with high sugar content. When you come to think of it, alkaline diet is not unusual for everyone especially when talking about a healthy diet.

Real Deal with Alkaline Diet

According to experts, acidic foods can decrease the pH of a person's urine. When the pH is abnormally low kidney stones tend to form. To counteract this situation a person needs to increase the pH through eating alkaline rich foods, that simple.

Since an alkaline diet means avoiding alcohol and any other foods with high acidity, it also means that you will decrease the risk of developing diseases associated with unhealthy diet like diabetes, hypertension, and obesity. Although no exact evidences can prove, some researchers have stated that alkaline diet can reduce the risk of cancer.

Things to Remember

In order for alkaline diet to work, you must condition yourself to adhere to the diet program. When it requires you to avoid unhealthy foods and drinks, then you better do it. Water therapy is an excellent alternative drink for soda and alcohol. In addition, so that you will not have a difficult time figuring out which are alkaline and which are acid foods, it is best that you make a list of each category. Perhaps you can research online on what foods are rich in alkaline and those having high acid content. Alkaline foods are not that hard to point because the majority of foods belong to vegetables and fruits classification.

WHAT AN ALKALINE DIET CAN DO

An alkaline diet is a nutritional plan that emphasizes fresh fruit, vegetables, tubers, nuts, roots and legumes as the main food source. An alkalizing diet is often called a raw food diet or a detox diet. This type of eating plan has become very popular as we have come to realize the incredible health benefits of certain types of raw foods.

Enjoying a diet high in alkaline food helps to keep the acidic levels in the body down. You can easily check your PH by using a PH strip first thing in the morning. PH levels below 7 is considered acidic and is detrimental to your health. A PH level of 7.3 to 7.45 is considered ideal for good health.

So why should you even care about this? Alkalizing is so important because the cells of the body function best in a slightly alkaline environment, while dangerous organisms such as cancers thrive in an acidic environment. Studies show that cancer cells are destroyed in a matter of hours when a body reaches a PH balance of 8.0!

The leading cause of osteoporosis? You guessed it, high acidic levels in the body usually caused by eating too much meat.

Foods that contribute to an acidic environment in the body include: dairy, meats, sugary snacks, caffeine, soda and processed foods. These are the types of foods most of usually eat throughout day, every day.

The best way to ensure you are enjoying a healthy, non-acidic diet is by getting most of your nutrition from fresh, live, organic foods. Spend at least two weeks eating nothing but high alkaline food, and then slowly begin to add back other foods and you will instantly see which foods work for you and which foods work against you. This type of eating is commonly called a detox diet because it flushes the acidic toxins out of the body.

Some great foods to enjoy during your detox include: avocado, cabbage, celery, dandelion, karmut grass, lettuce, sprouted radish, alfalfa grass, barley grass, cayenne pepper, cucumber, beans and so much more.

Foods that are very acidic and should be avoided include: beer, cheese, eggs, ketchup, pork, veal, white bread, ocean fish, liquor, pistachios and artificial sweeteners just to name a few.

Most people enjoy a miraculous shift in how the look and feel after only a few days on this type of diet plan. Raw food alkalizing diets are also great because food preparation is quick and easy; not to mention there is an endless variety of what you can enjoy on this type of diet.

THE ALKALINE DIET MYTH

The alkaline diet is also known as the acid-alkaline diet or the alkaline ash diet. It is based around the idea that the foods you eat leave behind an "ash" residue after they have been metabolized. This ash can be acid or alkaline.

Proponents of this diet claim that certain foods can affect the acidity and alkalinity of bodily fluids, including urine and blood. If you eat foods with an acidic ash, they make the body acidic. If you eat foods with an alkaline ash, they make the body alkaline.

Acid ash is thought to make you vulnerable to diseases such as cancer, osteoporosis, and muscle wasting, whereas alkaline ash is considered to be protective. To make sure you stay alkaline, it is recommended that you keep track of your urine using handy pH test strips.

For those who do not fully understand human physiology and are not nutrition experts, diet claims like this sounds rather convincing. However, is it really true? The following will debunk this myth and clear up some confusion regarding the alkaline diet.

But first, it is necessary to understand the meaning of the pH value.

Put simply, the pH value is a measure of how acidic or alkaline something is. The pH value ranges from 0 to 14.

- 0-7 is acidic

- 7 is neutral

7-14 is alkaline

For example, the stomach is loaded with highly acidic hydrochloric acid, a pH value between 2 and 3.5. The acidity helps kill germs and break down food.

On the other hand, the human blood is always slightly alkaline, with a pH of between 7.35 to 7.45. Normally, the body has several effective

mechanisms (discussed later) to keep the blood pH within this range. Falling out of it is very serious and can be fatal.

Effects Of Foods On Urine And Blood pH

Foods leave behind an acid or alkaline ash. Acid ash contains phosphate and sulfur. Alkaline ash contains calcium, magnesium, and potassium.

Certain food groups are considered acidic, neutral, or alkaline.

- Acidic: Meats, fish, dairy, eggs, grains, and alcohol.

- Neutral: Fats, starches, and sugars.

- Alkaline: Fruits, vegetables, nuts, and

legumes.

- Urine pH

Foods you eat change the pH of your urine. If you have a green smoothie for breakfast, your urine, in a few hours, will be more alkaline than if you had bacon and eggs.

For someone on an alkaline diet, urine pH can be very easily monitored and may even provide instant gratification. Unfortunately, urine pH is neither a good indicator of the overall pH of the body, nor is it a good indicator of general health.

Blood pH

Foods you eat do not change your blood pH. When you eat something with an acid ash like protein, the acids produced are quickly neutralized by bicarbonate ions in the blood. This reaction produces carbon dioxide, which is exhaled through the lungs, and salts, which are excreted by the kidneys in your urine.

During the process of excretion, the kidneys produce new bicarbonate ions, which are returned to the blood to replace the bicarbonate that was initially used to neutralize the acid. This creates a sustainable cycle in which the body is able to maintain the pH of the blood within a tight range.

Therefore, as long as your kidneys are functioning

normally, your blood pH will not be influenced by the foods you eat, whether they are acidic or alkaline. The claim that eating alkaline foods will make your body or blood pH more alkaline is not true.

Acidic Diet And Cancer

Those who advocate an alkaline diet claim that it can cure cancer because cancer can only grow in an acidic environment. By eating an alkaline diet, cancer cells cannot grow but die.

This hypothesis is very flawed. Cancer is perfectly capable of growing in an alkaline environment. In fact, cancer grows in normal body tissue which has a slightly alkaline pH of 7.4. Many experiments have confirmed this by successfully growing cancer cells in an alkaline environment.

However, cancer cells do grow faster with acidity. Once a tumor starts to develop, it creates its own acidic environment by breaking down glucose and reducing circulation. Therefore, it is not the acidic environment that causes cancer but the cancer that causes the acidic environment.

Even more interesting is a 2005 study by the National Cancer Institute which uses vitamin C (ascorbic acid) to treat cancer. They found that by administering pharmacologic doses intravenously, ascorbic acid successfully killed cancer cells without harming normal cells. This is another example of cancer cells being vulnerable to acidity, as opposed to alkalinity.

In short, there is no scientific link between eating an acidic diet and cancer. Cancer cells can grow in both acidic and alkaline environments.

Acidic Diet And Osteoporosis

Osteoporosis is a progressive bone disease characterized by a decrease in bone mineral content, leading to lowered bone density and strength and higher risk of a broken bone.

Proponents of the alkaline diet believe that in order to maintain a constant blood pH, the body takes alkaline minerals like calcium from the bones to neutralize the acids from an acidic diet. As discussed above, this is absolutely not true. The kidneys and the respiratory system are responsible for regulating blood pH, not the bones.

In fact, many studies have shown that increasing animal protein intake is positive for bone metabolism as it increases calcium retention and activates IGF-1 (insulin-like growth factor-1) that stimulates bone regeneration. Thus, the hypothesis that an acidic diet causes bone loss is not supported by science.

Acidic Diet And Muscle Wasting

Advocates of the alkaline diet believe that in order to eliminate excess acid caused by an acidic diet, the kidneys will steal amino acids (building blocks of protein) from muscle tissues, leading to muscle loss. The proposed mechanism is similar to the one causing osteoporosis.

As discussed, blood pH is regulated by the kidneys and the lungs, not the muscles. Hence, acidic foods like meats, dairy, and eggs do not cause muscle loss. As a matter of fact, they are complete dietary proteins that will support muscle repair and help prevent muscle wasting.

What Did Our Ancestors Eat?

A number of studies have examined whether our pre-agricultural ancestors ate net acidic or net alkaline diets. Very interestingly, they found that about half of the hunter-gatherers ate net acid-forming diets, while the other half ate net alkaline-forming diets.

Acid-forming diets were more common as people moved further north of the equator. The less hospitable the environment, the more animal proteins they ate. In more tropical environments where fruits and vegetables were abundant, their diet became more alkaline.

From an evolutionary perspective, the theory that acidic or protein-rich diets cause diseases like cancer, osteoporosis, and muscle loss is not valid. Half of the hunter-gatherers were eating net acid-forming diets, yet, they had no evidence of such degenerative diseases.

It is worth noting that there is no one-size-fits-all diet that works for everyone, which is why Metabolic Typing is so helpful in determining your optimal diet. Due to our genetic variances, some people will benefit from an acidic diet, some an alkaline diet, and some in between. Thus the saying: one man's food can be another man's poison.

Final Thoughts

It is true that many people who have switched to an alkaline diet see significant health improvements. However, do bear in mind that other reasons may be at work:

Most of us do not eat enough vegetables and fruits. According to the Center for Disease and Prevention, only 9% of Americans eat enough vegetables and 13% enough fruits. If you switch to an alkaline diet, you are automatically eating more vegetables and fruits. After all, they are very rich in phytochemicals, antioxidants, and fiber which are essential to good health. When you eat more vegetables and fruits, you are probably eating less processed foods too.

Eating less dairy and eggs will benefit those who are lactose-intolerant or have a food sensitivity to eggs, which is rather common among the general population.

Eating less grains will benefit those who are gluten-sensitive or have leaky gut or an autoimmune disease.

Alkaline Water

One last point worth mentioning is that many people believe that drinking alkaline water (pH of 9.5 vs. pure water's pH of 7.0.) is healthier based on similar reasoning as the alkaline diet. Anyhow, it is not true. Water that is too alkaline can be detrimental to your health and lead to nutritional disequilibrium.

If you drink alkaline water all the time, it will neutralize your stomach acid and raise the alkalinity of your stomach. Over time, it will impair your ability to digest food and absorb nutrients and minerals. With less acidity in the stomach, it will also open the door for bacteria and parasites to get into your small intestine.

The bottom line is that alkaline water is not the answer to good health. Do not be fooled by marketing gimmicks. Instead, invest in a good water filtration system for your home. Clean, filtered water is still the best water for your body.

THE ALKALINE DIET: A LITTLE-KNOWN AND POWERFUL WEIGHT LOSS PLAN

What if you knew about a weight loss program that would help you lose weight and feel younger? Would you try it? The alkaline diet and lifestyle has been around for over 60 years, yet many people aren't familiar with its natural, safe and proven weight loss properties!

The alkaline diet is not a gimmick or a fad. It's a healthy and easy way to enjoy new levels of health. In this post you'll learn about what this dietary plan is, what makes it different, and how it can produce life- changing results for you, your waistline and your health.

Are you enjoying a slim and sexy body today? If so, you're in the minority.

Sadly, over 65 percent of Americans are either overweight or obese. If you're overweight, you probably experience symptoms of ill-health like fatigue, swelling, sore joints, and a host of other signs of poor health.

Worse yet, you probably feel like giving up on ever enjoying the body you want and deserve. Perhaps you've been told that you're just getting older, but that simply isn't the truth. Don't buy into that lie. Other cultures have healthy, lean seniors who enjoy great health into their nineties!

The truth is, your body is a brilliantly designed machine and if you have any symptoms of ill-health this is a sure sign that your body's chemistry is too acidic. Your symptoms are just a cry for help. This is because the body doesn't just break down one day. Instead, your health erodes slowly over time, finally falling into 'dis-ease'.

What's wrong with the way you're eating now?

The Standard American Diet (S.A.D.) focuses on refined carbohydrates, sugars, alcohol, meats and dairy. These foods are all highly acid- forming. Meanwhile, despite pleas from the nutritional experts, we

simply don't eat enough of the alkalizing foods such as fresh fruits, veggies, nuts, and legumes.

In short, our S.A.D. lifestyle upsets the natural acid-alkaline balance our bodies need. This condition causes obesity, low-level aches and pains, colds and flu, and eventually disease sets in.

We've lost our way. This is where an alkaline diet can help restore our health.

I'm sure you're familiar with the term pH, which refers to the level of acidity or alkalinity contained in something. Alkalinity is measured on a scale. You can take a simple and inexpensive test at home to see where your alkalinity level falls, as well as to monitor it regularly.

Medical researchers and scientists have known for at least 70 years this lesser-known fact....your body requires a certain pH level, or delicate balance of your body's acid-alkaline levels - for optimal health and vitality.

You might think..."I don't need to know all this chemistry. Besides, what does the proper pH balance and alkalinity matter to me?" I know these were my questions when I first heard about alkaline eating.

We'll use two examples of how acid and alkalinity plays a role in your body.

1. We all know that our stomach has acid in it. Along with enzymes, this acid is essential for breaking food into basic elements that can be absorbed by the digestive tract. What if we didn't have any acid in our stomachs? We would die from malnutrition in no time because the body couldn't utilize a whole piece of meat or a whole piece of anything, for that matter! Make sense?

2. Different parts of our body require different levels of acidity or alkalinity. For example, your blood requires a slightly more alkaline level than your stomach acids. What if your

blood was too acidic? It would virtually eat through your veins and arteries, causing a massive internal hemorrhage!

While these examples demonstrate that the various parts or systems in the body need different pH levels, we don't need to worry about that.

Our problem is simple and it's this.....we are simply to acidic overall, period. If you're interested in learning more about pH you can find tons of information on the web by simply searching the term.

The most important thing to know is this. When your body is too acidic over a long time, it leads to many diseases like obesity, arthritis, bone density loss, high blood pressure, heart disease and stroke. The list is endless, because the body simply gives up the battle for vitality and goes into survival mode as long as it can.

An alkaline diet is unique.

Many diets focus on the same foods that cause you to be overweight or sick in the first place. They simply ask you to eat less of those things, to eat more time per day, or to combine them differently.

In fairness to these diet's creators, they know that many of us don't want to make the bigger changes for our health. We like a diet that's focused on processed and refined foods, our meat, our sugar, alcohols and such. The diet creators are simply trying to help us make easier changes.

We've gotten used to eating this way, and it's not ALL our fault! Greedy food processing giants have a vested interest in keeping us eating this way. Profits are much higher in this sector of the food industry than in the production of your more basic foods like fruits and veggies.

So, again, YES...this diet is different. If those other diets worked you would you would be feeling lean, healthy and vital you wouldn't need to read this article. You wouldn't need a dietary change.

- Here's a partial list of foods that you can eat freely in an alkaline diet:

- Fresh fruits and freshly made juices

- Fresh veggies and juices

- Cooked veggies

- Some legumes and soy

- Lean proteins and some eggs

- Certain grains

- Healthy fats and nuts

*You may be surprised to learn that some veggies and fruits are better for you than others!

You can consume limited quantities of these foods and beverages:

- Dairy

- Many common grains

- Refined foods and sugars

- Alcohol and caffeine

What's it like to be on the alkaline diet, and what results can you expect?

Like any change in diet or lifestyle, you'll go through an adjustment period. Yet because you're burning the cleanest fuel, which your body craves, so unlike many diet plans, you won't ever need to feel hungry. Plus, you can eat all you like until you're satisfied. You also won't need to count calories. And you'll enjoy plenty of variety, so you'll never get bored with eating.

Think of an alkaline diet as a type of 'juice fast' for the body. Only it's not so extreme. You're eating nutrient-dense, easily digestible foods that your body craves. When you provide all the cells of the body that it so desperately needs, your hunger goes away. And there's no need to worry about boring veggies, since there are tons of delicious recipes found on the web and in books.

With all the diet plans out there, why should you consider an alternative plan like the alkaline diet?

When followed properly, you can expect to melt the fat away more easily than with traditional plans. Many testimonials exist where people report losing over two pounds each week. (And that much weight wouldn't be

wise in most diet programs.) Plus your skin will become more supple again, your energy will increase and you'll feel younger.

Plus, the alkaline diet does two important things that traditional diets

don't.

1. It provides superior nourishment to your body's cells.

2. It naturally helps to detoxify and cleanse the cells, too.

These two facts are behind the reason why an alkaline diet work so

quickly and safely.

One, final note, when considering an alkaline diet. Since it's can be quite different from the way you may be used to eating, you might wonder if you can return to your former eating habits. The honest answer is that it's smart to continue as many of the principles as you can once you have lost all your weight. But it doesn't need to be all or nothing. Anything you do to adopt a healthier diet will greatly increase your chances for keeping the weight off for good.

ACID TO ALKALINE DIET, HOW TO LOSE WEIGHT AND LIVE A HEALTHIER LIFESTYLE NATURALLY

Acid to Alkaline Diet

The acid to alkaline diet is becoming a more talked about subject nowadays but still the majority of the population are unaware of what it is. People who die young, have health problems, suffer from obesity etc., generally have a very acidic internal environment whereas people who live to a very old age and don't suffer from serious health problems have an internal environment that is more alkaline in nature.

In the modern Western world the vast majority of people live a very unhealthy lifestyle, predominantly eating junk and unhealthy food and being constantly exposed to other factors that drastically impact our health in a negative way, in drastic contrast to the acid to alkaline diet. According to the World Health Organization (WHO), there are more that one billion obese adults world-wide, with around 300 million of them clinically obese. This statistic is scary and is dramatically increasing everyday!

As a health care practitioner myself, people often ask

me what are the best ways to stay healthy. I often tell my patients that in order for us to live a healthy life, not be over weight, avoid serious disease and illnesses and generally live to a good old age with vitality and vigour, it is essential that we pay attention to the acid to alkaline diet. By observing your bodies pH levels and eating accordingly to ensure your body is more alkaline than acidic, people experience things like rapid weight loss (by an accelerated fat disposal process), they will live longer, feel less stressed, have an improved immune system, get better and more restful sleep, have more energy and can also experience an increase in libido. These benefits alone are of course of tremendous importance to health, longevity and a happy life. By allowing the body to detox in this way through the acid to alkaline diet people also have an increased ability to absorb vitamins and minerals and help avoid many nasty diseases including cancer and arthritis. With a more alkaline body,

stress and pressure on the internal organs is eased, skin, bones and cells regenerate and help keep you youthful.

Conversely, if a person's body is too acidic they can easily experience obesity by gaining and holding onto fat, they will age quicker, a lack of energy will be common, they will easily and consistently attract disease and virus' and create an internal environment where yeast and bacteria can easily thrive.

The majority of people living in the Western world don't follow an acid to alkaline diet and are generally more on the acidic scale. This is due largely to our diet. Eating things like junk food, burgers, fizzy drinks, having a high sugar intake, fried foods, unnatural fruit juices, imitation foods, energy drinks and processed foods for example, all push our bodies internal environment down on the acidic scale. There are even some otherwise healthy foods to be aware of, strawberries, mangos and peaches for example are very high in sugar, therefore create an acidic environment in the body. Some other surprises that also cause acidic build up include rice, tuna, oats and cheese, so these foods are to be limited when following an acid to alkaline diet. This is one reason why it is very important to know exactly what foods will cause an acid reaction and which will make you more alkaline. Other considerations that also cause our bodies to be more acidic include various chemicals, tobacco, radiation, pesticides, artificial sweeteners, air pollution, alcohol, drugs and stress.

Optimal pH to get all the benefits from alkalinity is 7.4pH. If your body goes 3-4 points either way you will die! The pH scale is as follows:

- 0 = total acid/battery acid, hydrochloric acid

- 1 = gastric juices

- 2 = vinegar

- 3 = beer

- 4 = wine, tomato juice

- 5 = rain

- 6 = milk

- 7 = pure water

- 8 = sea water

- 9 = baking soda

- 10 = detergent, milk of magnesia

- 11 = ammonia, lime water

- 12 = bleach

- 13 = lye

- 14 = Total Alkaline/Sodium Hydroxide

The acid to alkaline diet will help your body stay at the optimal range, around 7.4pH. The bodies reaction to trying to keep this acid, alkaline balance is both incredible and fascinating. When your body is too acidic it tries everything to get to a more alkaline state. When this happens the body stores some acid in your fat to keep it from doing harm to our body which is a good thing, but your body then holds on to the fat for protection, causing the person to put on weight.

When there is excess acid internally, the body finds alkaline elsewhere from your bones and teeth but your bones and teeth get so drained that they become frail and start to decay. This can lead to many diseases of the bones and teeth including arthritis and tooth decay. This would not happen if a person were following an acid to alkaline diet.

The build up of acid generally will settle away from your healthier organs but instead it gravitates towards your weakest organs that are already prone to disease. It's like a pack of wolves looking for the weakest amongst the herd, picking off the easy prey. As your weaker organs are targeted it makes it much easier for serious diseases to set in, including cancer. It is important to realise that cancer cells become dormant if you are at 7.4pH (which is the bodies optimum pH levels), thus further underlining the importance of maintaining a healthy pH level in our bodies by following the acid to alkaline diet.

When there is acid in the system it also contaminates your blood stream. This in turn prevents the bloods ability to deliver oxygen to the tissues. RBC's are surrounded by a negative charge so they can bounce off each other and move around in the blood very quickly and deliver their goodness.

But when you are too acidic they lose their negative charge and they stick together, causing them to move very slowly. This causes them to struggle to deliver nutrients and oxygen in our system. One of the first symptoms of this poisoning is you start to feel a loss of energy even though you are getting enough sleep. Starting an acid to alkaline diet can correct this very quickly. Your blood also has this reaction after drinking alcohol.

Let's put all this into perspective; it takes about 33 glasses of water to neutralize one glass of coke! I'm not even going to mention here what it takes to neutralize some of the other things that we are putting into our bodies, I think you get the picture!

One great way to consistently make your body more alkaline is by having green drinks everyday. They are very easy to make, taste great and are packed with vitamins, minerals and chlorophyll which fuel our body. Chlorophyll is a big part of the acid to alkaline diet and is the green blood of plants. It is a very powerful detoxifyer, blood builder, cleaner and oxygen booster. In fact, the benefits of chlorophyll on our bodies are far too numerous to include in this article. There are many recipes for making tasty green drinks. The one I am currently having everyday is as follows; 2 apples, 4 sticks celery, 1/3 cucumber, big handful of baby spinach leaves and one avocado. I have been doing this everyday (more or less) for about the last six months and not once have I been sick. I have also noticed an increase in energy and I am also benefiting from more restful sleep.

IS ALKALINE WATER EXTRA HEALTHY OR JUST A HOAX☐

Alkaline water is selling incredibly well. Its sales jumped from $47 million in 2014 to a whopping $427 million in 2017. Marketers claim that alkaline water can energize and detoxify the body, and lead to superior hydration. Not only that, it can also correct acidity in your tissues, which can then prevent or reverse cancer, arthritis, osteoporosis, and other degenerative diseases.

Regrettably, there is virtually no rigorous scientific evidence that can back up such health claims. As a matter of fact, it may be harmful to drink this water on a regular basis. The following explains what alkaline water is and why it is impossible to achieve what marketers claim it can do in the body.

What Is Alkaline Water?

The concept of acidity or alkalinity of the body or of water is based on the pH scale. The pH scale goes from 0 to 14 and a pH of 7 is neutral. Anything with a pH below 7 is considered acidic and anything with a pH above 7 is alkaline.

The acronym "pH" is short for "potential of hydrogen". pH is a measure of the concentration of hydrogen ions. The lower the pH, the more free hydrogen ions it has. The higher the pH, the fewer free hydrogen ions it has. One pH unit reflects a tenfold change in ion concentration, so there are 10 times as many hydrogen ions available at a pH of 7 than at a pH of 8.

Our blood is slightly alkaline, with a pH of 7.4. Pure water has a neutral pH of 7, while natural water ranges from around 6.5 to 8.5 depending on surrounding soil and vegetation, seasonal variations, and weather.

Bottled waters marketed as being alkaline typically claim to have a pH between 8 and 10. Some are from springs or artesian wells that are naturally alkaline because of dissolved alkalizing compounds such as calcium, magnesium, potassium, silica, and bicarbonate. Others are

transformed by a process called electrolysis that separates the water into alkaline and acid fractions. There are also expensive water ionizing machines marketed for home use.

Origin Of The Alkaline Diet

The marketing claims behind alkaline water are based on an old idea called the acid-ash hypothesis. It says that eating certain acidic foods like meats, dairy, and eggs results in something called acid ash in the body, which increases your acid levels and causes adverse health effects.

In 2002, an alternative medicine practitioner called Robert O. Young turned the acid-ash hypothesis into a fad alkaline diet with a popular series of books called the pH Miracle. According to his books, an alkaline diet could treat all sorts of illnesses, from poor digestion to cancer. So far, no rigorous research studies have been able to back up the health claims behind the alkaline diet. In 2017, Young was sentenced to three years in jail for practicing medicine without a license.

Why Alkaline Water Cannot Turn The Body Alkaline

Marketers claim that their special water can turn the body alkaline. The truth is that they do not even understand the basic chemistry of how the human body works!

The main reason why drinking alkaline water cannot produce the health benefits claimed by the marketers is because one simply cannot alter the pH of the blood or the body this way.

Our diet, including the water we drink and the medications and supplements we take, can only alter the pH of our urine. Home test kits to measure the pH of urine do not relay any information about the body's pH at all.

The lungs and kidneys are the organs that regulate the body's pH, which is always kept in a very narrow range because all our enzymes are designed to work at pH 7.4. Even a small fluctuation, as little as 0.05 in

our blood, can become life-threatening. That is why patients with kidney disease and lung dysfunction often rely on dialysis machines and mechanical ventilators respectively to avoid even a small disruption of pH balance in the blood.

In the stomach, where stomach acid is secreted, the pH is 1.5 to 3.5. It is a very acidic environment because the acid is necessary to break down the food and to kill all the germs and bacteria that may be in our food.

When we drink alkaline water and it comes in contact with the very acidic stomach, it is immediately neutralized because alkaline water has no buffers. A buffer is a chemical that can react with small amounts of either acid or alkaline substance to prevent changes in pH. An example of an alkaline buffer is baking soda (or sodium bicarbonate). Our lungs use bicarbonate as a pH-stabilizing buffer to maintain a constant blood pH.

Marketers claim that as the stomach acid neutralizes the alkaline water, bicarbonate ions are released into the blood, resulting in an alkalizing effect. This could only be true if the alkaline water effectively neutralized all the stomach acid, like baking soda would have done. But in reality, it is impossible for alkaline water to neutralize any significant quantity of stomach acid to create this "net alkalizing effect". As it happens, it is the other way around, the stomach acid completely neutralizes the alkaline water!

Alkaline Foods And Cancer

Proponents of an alkaline diet and marketers of alkaline water believe that overly acidic diets cause the body to become too acidic, which increases your risk of cancer. Although it is true that the immediate environment around cancer cells can be acidic, do know that it is due to differences in the way tumors create energy and use oxygen as compared to healthy tissues, not the acidic foods (such as meats, dairy, and eggs) that you eat.

Similarly, understand that their proposed answer to increase your intake of healthier alkaline foods like vegetables, fruits, and alkaline water can do nothing to change your body's pH. Veggies are good for you but for a different reason - they are high in vitamins, minerals, and antioxidants which are anti-inflammatory and cancer-protective.

Alkaline Water For Detoxification And Hydration

Initial health improvements reported by people who drink this type of water can be attributed to the simple fact that they are drinking more water, resulting in improved hydration and detoxification. There is the placebo effect as well.

Moreover, alkaline water may contain higher mineral concentration, which is known to have beneficial health effects, especially when one's diet consists of mainly processed or junk foods that are very low in nutrients.

Final Word

Keep in mind that drinking too much highly alkaline water on a regular basis may not be a good thing. It may lower the stomach pH and compromise digestion. For people who already have insufficient stomach acid production, it may even allow bacteria or other harmful organisms to survive.

For individuals who have a kidney condition or are taking medication that alters their kidney function, the minerals in alkaline water can start to accumulate in their bodies.

However, if you are suffering from acid reflux, the alkalinity may give you some degree of short-term relief the same way TUMS or other antacids that contain alkaline ions will do though neither addresses the root cause of your problem.

RULES FOR A PH BALANCED DIET

There are four elementary principles for selecting foods to ensure the proper quantities of acidifying, alkalizing, and acid foods in the diet. These are accompanied by four additional rules to be followed by people who are unable to metabolize acids properly.

Rule one: A meal should never consist solely of acidifying foods but should always contain alkaline foods.

A meal of meat with pasta, or fish and rice, with cake and coffee for dessert is not a recommended menu because it consists entirely of acidifying foods; the same applies to a meatless meal of pasta with tomato sauce followed by a dessert sweetened with white sugar. By adding vegetables to this meal in the form of salads or raw or cooked vegetables, the alkaline intake at least partially compensates for the acids. Vegetables are typically included with meals, but often in such small quantities that their effect is negligible.

Rule two: The amount of alkalizing foods should be greater proportionately than the amount of acidifying foods at anyone meal.

The proportion of foods that produce alkaline elements should always be greater than that of foods that produce acids. Eating in this manner ensures that the acids are neutralized at the intestinal or tissue level without any need for the body to draw from its reserves.

Rule three: The proportion of alkalizing foods should be even greater proportionately when there is pronounced acidification of the internal environment or when the individual is unable to metabolize acids properly.

The more the body is weakened or exhausted, the less alkaline reserve it has for its buffer system, and the less capable it is of oxidizing acids. Putting less acid into the body makes it easier for the body to maintain its acid-alkaline balance.

Rule four: A diet consisting solely of alkaline vegetables and plant- based food is possible, but only for a limited period (one to two weeks).

An exclusively alkaline diet, consisting solely of vegetables, potatoes, bananas, almonds, and so forth, cannot be continued indefinitely because it is seriously inadequate in protein. Such diets are useful when acidification is very significant and the disorders it has caused are acute, intense, and painful. The abrupt, complete elimination of all acids allows the body to recover more rapidly and return to a normal acid-alkaline balance. An exclusively alkaline diet should remain a short-term therapeutic action so as not to compromise health.

There are four additional rules that people suffering from an inability to metabolize acids properly should heed.

Rule five: A meal should never consist solely of acid foods but should always include alkaline foods.

This rule is almost identical to rule one, but it involves acid rather than acidifying foods. Eating fruits and yogurt exclusively or drinking only whey-based beverages is strongly discouraged, as the acid intake from such a diet is not compensated by any alkaline food, which forces the body to draw these substances from its own tissues. The risk of health problems caused by mineral depletion is therefore quite significant. These manifest as a sudden drop in vitality, the feeling that one's teeth are on edge, a chilly sensation, itching, joint pains, and others that have been discussed previously.

Alkaline foods that are good accompaniments to fresh fruits are fresh (unripened) cheeses, soft white cheese (large-curd cottage cheese, low- fat cream cheese, ricotta, quark, mozzarella, farmer cheese, fresh goat cheese, yogurt cheese), cream, almonds, bananas, salad greens, or a blend of raw fruits and vegetables.

Rule six: The quantities of acid and acidifying foods a person eats should be tailored to meet their personal metabolic capabilities.

The inability to metabolize acids properly is rarely absolute; it varies according to individual physiology as well as circumstances (such as stress, fatigue, work, and vacations). Each person has a certain rate at which he or she can metabolize acids properly, a rate that cannot be surpassed without overtaxing the body's capacity.

As long as the quantity of acids ingested or created by the digestion of food is below these rates, the body manages to neutralize them through oxidation before any of the health problems created by acidification manifest. Accordingly, for certain extremely sensitive individuals, half a golden apple no more-suits them just fine, but even a quarter of a Winesap apple is more than they can handle. For any given person, a certain quantity of a food can be acidifying, yet alkalizing or neutral in a lesser amount.

So if you have difficulty metabolizing acids, you can safely eat acid foods as long as you tailor the amount you consume to your physical capacities. Your tolerance threshold can also change over time. You can discover and keep track of your own threshold through experimentation and observation.

Rule seven: Acid foods should not be eaten too rapidly

An individual with an inability to metabolize acids properly, but with a normal acid-alkaline balance, can generally handle a sudden increase in acid intake (from eating a large quantity of fruit, for example) by drawing from the body's reserves, provided that this kind of event is the exception and not the rule. In fact, if the withdrawal of alkaline substances from the body's reserves is a unique event, the acid-alkaline balance is not endangered, and no acidification problem will occur.

But some time will have to go by before the body's reserves are replenished. If eating another piece of fruit puts additional acids into the body too soon, it has to draw from its already diminished reserves, which may not contain enough alkaline substances to neutralize the acid from the fruit, and acid-alkaline balance is compromised. Health problems due to acidification will appear not because the body was not intrinsically capable of neutralizing this fruit's acid-it had successfully

done so before-but because the fruit had been eaten too soon after the first fruit had been consumed.

By spacing out the ingestion of these hard-to-metabolize foods, you can increase your personal level of tolerance for them. This is useful to know, as it allows you to expand the selection of foods you can safely eat.

Rule eight: Acid foods must be eaten when the body is ready to receive

them.

There is an Arabic proverb that says: "Oranges are like

gold in the morning, silver at noon, and lead in the evening." For people with an inability to metabolize acids properly, the opposite is true. Oranges and fruits in general are harmful in the morning and much more beneficial at noon or in the evening. The reason for this is that by noon the body's "organic motor" has had the time to warm up and is turning over naturally. In fact, some people take a long time physically to wake up in the morning. The heart beats more slowly, blood pressure is low, and cellular exchanges-including oxidation-take place in slow motion. The body reaches cruising speed only after several hours of activity and a meal or two. If such a person eats fruits or drinks a glass of orange juice in the morning, not only will he or she have difficulty metabolizing the acids but, because the body is still working below its real capacity, it will have even greater trouble oxidizing acids than it normally would.

Along the same lines of reasoning, acids foods are metabolized better in the summer, when the weather is hot and sunny, as well as when one is rested (as opposed to feeling tired).

WHAT IS AN ALKALINE LIFESTYLE□

If you can remember back to your days in Chemistry 101, you learned the concept of alkaline and acid. There is a pH scale from 0 to 14. Pure acid is 0 and 14 is pure alkaline. So things like battery acid would be a

1 and Sodium hydroxide would be a 14. It takes 20 parts of acid to neutralize one part of alkaline. One number that we are all aware of is our body's temperature. It is around 98.6 degrees. There is another number that most people are not aware of. That number is 7.36. That is the pH level of our blood. Unlike our body temperature, our blood has to keep that constant rate or we would enter a condition called acidosis. Acidosis is a condition in which there is excessive acid in the body fluids. The acid would eventually burn holes in our arteries and we would die.

So why does all this matter to us? To answer that, I have to use the following saying, "We are what we eat." If I can add to that saying, I would say, we are also what we think. I will explain that in a bit. Let's start with what we consume. All foods have different minerals in them which make them fall somewhere in the 0 to 14 pH level. For example, take a good old can of Coke. The pH level is about 3.4 on the scale. It is very acidic. Asparagus is about 8.5. It is Very alkaline. So when you eat these foods, the stomach starts to digest the food and the vitamins, minerals and acids start to be absorbed in the stomach, with most of the nutrients being absorbed in the small intestine. Now, our bodies need to absorb some acid. Without it, we would not be healthy. Unfortunately, we consume a typical Western diet that is very highly acidic. We drink coffee and soda all day. We constantly test our body's ability to get rid of all this acid. Your body tries to keep up by using the alkalinity in the foods we eat. That is where the problem lies. We eat very little alkaline foods. If your body does not get it from our foods, your body will take it from the alkaline reserves that we store in our body fluids. If that becomes depleted, your body will start to steal from your calcium based organs like your bones and brain. Sounds bad, doesn't it. You would be correct.

If all this fails, your body keeps trying to fight back. It starts to produce

massive amounts of Cholesterol to surround the acid and remove it from

your blood stream. And by the way, I thought I would add that it takes that acid as far away from the internal organs as possible. Places like the Hips, butt, thighs, stomach and the back of your arms become the final resting place. Your blood vessels can only remove so much of the acid. After a while, Cholesterol starts to accumulate on the side of the walls and forms plaque. As the acid builds up in your blood, it starts to attack the blood cells. These cells have a positive charge on the inside and a negative charge on the outside. If your cells are healthy, the negative charges are pushing other cells away. It is very much like putting 2 magnets that are negatively charged together. They repel each other and flow freely. The acid starts to strip the negative charge away from the cell and they start to attract to each other. This is what they call blot clotting. You start to feel lethargic and tired all the time. The clots keep much needed oxygen from flowing through the system. The clot grows and eventually finds its way to the heart or your brain. That can spell lights out.

If all of that is not bad enough, we have the concept of disease. The wonderful world of germs. We have been told that germs cause sickness. Louis Pasteur was to thank for that. I am writing a blog entry that will put a kybosh on that theory. Let me give you an analogy. Have you ever been to the city dump? Well, if you have, one thing that you will see other that the endless trash is thousands of rats. These rats feed off the food and waste. They multiply at a feverous rate. They break the food down, but create their own waste in the process. Your body works in the same way. Look at the acidic environment in your body as the trash and the rats are equivalent to the germs.

The germs try to break the acid down. They too start to multiply and create their own waste. The environment gets worse and worse.

Let's throw some common sense into the mix here. If we had a problem of rats or mice in our house, what would we do? We would spread poison or set traps to kill the rodents. That would work for a while, but what would happen? They would eventual come back. Why? Because we took care of the problem, but not the cause. The problem is the rats, but the cause is the trash and mess that we have at the house. Here is a novel idea. Why not get rid of the trash and mess? Hmmmm. No mess, no rats. Modern medicine works like the rat principle. They try to kill the

rats with procedures and drugs. Those rats just keep coming back. The problem is the rats bring their vulture buddies to join in on the feast.

I know you are staying to yourself, "What do I do?" The answer is to take care of the cause and get rid of the trash. It is that simple. Disease cannot live in an healthy alkaline body. It can however live in an acidic environment. There are several ways to become more alkaline. Today we are going to focus on food and drink. The first things we have to do are learn what foods are acidic and what foods are alkaline. Before I go any further, I am going to ask you to be open and to not discount what I am going to say. Just take in what I say and then do your own homework. Don't just take my word for it. This is where change comes in. We all just love to change. Yea right...

You will notice this about the list. On the acidic side, you have Meats, dairy, seafood, and sugar. On the Alkaline side, you have vegetable, some fruits, grains, and legumes. So what are you saying? Should I become a vegetarian? No I am not saying that. Currently, most people have an 80/20 diet. 80% acidic and 20% alkaline. I am just telling you to flip that. Eat 80% alkaline and 20% acidic. I will tell you this. When I first saw this, my answer was probably the same as yours. I said to myself, "There is NO WAY I could do this". I ate meat for breakfast, lunch, and dinner. I drank Coffee all day. I ate so much cheese, they called me Fedda. Fetty/Fedda, Get it? Anyway, my answer was to transition my toxic diet to a healthy one very slowly. I started to introduce more alkaline vegetables to my diet and reduced the acidic ones. It did not take long for me to get to the 80/20. My cravings for acidic foods just faded away.

So why did I do this in the first place?

In a few words, I was a mess. My weight was starting to get out of control. My health was starting to dwindle. I had bad headaches, horrible reflux disease, my joints were sore and cracking when I got up or went up the stairs. I was dealing with sinus problems, allergies and lower back pain. I was always tired. I was depressed and taking depression medication. I was always fighting off acne, colds and all types of sickness. You're not supposed to have acne at 40. I needed to

do something and I felt like I needed to do it fast. I am the kind of person that will devour information on a subject. I set out to learn how to be healthy. My goals were easy. It had to be common sense. I did not want to go on a diet, and it had to be from God.

Since I was always into fitness, it did not take me long to accomplish my goals. After I reached an alkaline way of living, I started to notice my issues fading away. For a few months I was eating 100% alkaline foods. I was starting to lose weight at about 2 pounds a day. I lost 45 pounds in no time. I even started to worry that I was going to waste away to nothing. That did not happen. I stopped at about 180 and have been there ever since. All my pains and problems are gone. I don't get sick. I don't take any medication. I feel wonderful. I will admit that it was a little tough in the beginning. I was not a big vegetable eater. My tastes have changed drastically. I have no cravings for the sugar laden processed foods. I will never go back. I have more energy and stamina. I feel better now than I did when I was twenty. My suggestion to you is to try this for a month. After a month I am willing to bet that you will never go back.

People ask me if I cheat at all. Of course I do. I am not fanatical about this. I do not stress about what I eat. Stress creates more acid in your body. More than any food you could eat. If I want to have a cup of coffee or a piece of cake every once in a while I will. Also keep in mind, people will look at you funny. You will not be the norm. It is a shame that being sick, overweight, and popping pills have become normal. God gave me this body to take care of. In the bible, it says that our bodies are the temple of the Holy Spirit. I can at least give the spirit a clean place to live.

ALKALINE FOODS - ACID FOODS - THE 80/20 ACID ALKALINE RATIO

Many of us get so caught up in eating to look good that we often forget to stick to the basics and focus on our health. Without our health in line, we won't ever achieve that dream physique anyways so it is always best to focus on health first.

Our typical mode of focusing on the outward physique and less on our insides tends to ruin most attempts for a stronger, leaner, healthier body. Out of all of the processes essential to a head turning physique, a well functioning body is likely the most important and neglecting your health at the expense of a temporary gain is a recipe for sure failure.

In order to keep your body functioning at its peak you must make sure that all of the processes involved aren't overloaded with toxins and overwhelmed by bad lifestyle choices.

Most of us do not live the right way, we eat the wrong foods, we don't get enough sleep, we are stressed out, and we don't get enough fresh air. With all off the abuse we put our bodies through, we can't expect it to function how it's supposed to.

It is funny how most of us get so frustrated when our

bodies do not respond how we want them to when all we have to do is just listen to what the body needs. Similar to a high performance race car, the human body must be given the proper fuel, maintenance, and service in order to ensure high performance and longevity. If we take care of the body, the body will take care of the rest.

Today I want to discuss the acid / alkaline balance and how maintaining the proper balance can help you improve your health, well being, and get leaner faster.

First the basics. Water has a pH (measured according to the potential of hydrogen scale) of 7.0. This range is considered neutral, as water is neither alkaline or acid. Any substance with a pH greater than 7.0 is

alkaline, and any substance with a pH lower than 7.0 is acidic. For a human to maintain a proper balance, it is best to shoot for a range between 6.0 and 6.8.

The acid-alkaline balance of the blood must be stabilized via the food we eat and, as such, we must give the body a constant supply of potassium, magnesium, calcium, and sodium because these important minerals help neutralize the acid wastes that accumulate when we consume proteins, sugars, and starches.

Acid wastes can also be especially dangerous because they are believed to cause a variety of health problems and chronic diseases.

If you have suffered with chronic symptoms such as water retention, migraines, low blood pressure, insomnia, sunken eyes, bad breath, tooth sensitivity to acidic fruits, and/or alternating diarrhea and constipation you may be suffering from acidosis. This term (acidosis) means that your body chemistry is likely imbalanced and overly acidic.

Various changes within the body can also throw off the natural acid balance, which can cause an acidic surge in body fluids and cause metabolic acidosis. Various disorders and diseases like stomach ulcers, obesity, kidney disease, liver problems, anorexia, adrenal disorders, diabetes, and fever can rob the body of its natural alkaline base, but typically, a bad diet plays the key role in creating an acidic environment within the body.

Note: Studies have shown that the over consumption of aspirin and vitamin C can also deplete the natural alkaline base.

When training to build a great physique, we so often get caught up in eating proteins and trying to build lean muscle, that in the process we disrupt the natural acid/alkaline balance in the body and become overly acidic.

It is hard to train and recover effectively when suffering with the annoying effects of acidosis.

As I mentioned earlier, proteins are acid forming foods and we must eat alkaline forming foods to neutralize the acid wastes from protein consumption. This means that you should probably be eating a bunch more veggies with that chicken breast than you usually do.

Finding a perfect balance can be challenging and confusing at first, but a good way to approach it is to try to maintain an 80% alkaline and 20% acid ratio. That means that in order to maintain a healthy, balanced pH, you need to eat a diet that consists of 80% alkaline forming foods and 20% acid forming foods.

Proteins and starches are acid, vegetables and fruits are alkaline. Just about all of the metabolic wastes of the body are acids so we need to eat alkaline forming foods like fruits and vegetables to help neutralize these acid wastes.

Recent studies have shown that the average American diet only consists of about 15-20% fruits and vegetables. This means that most people in this country are getting the majority of their calories from acid forming foods. In light of the current health crisis in America, I think that it is safe to say that there is a strong correlation between acidosis and disease.

For optimal health, fruits and vegetables should make up 80% of your diet. Starches and proteins should make up the last 20%. This guarantees your diet will be 80% alkaline and 20% acid.

Here is a list that outlines the foods that are alkaline and the foods that are acid.

Table 1.0 Alkaline Forming Foods

---Vegetables---

- Artichokes

- Broccoli

- Cabbage

- Cauliflower

- Celery

- Cucumber

- Green Beans

- Kudzu

- Lettuce

- Mushrooms

- Onion

- Radish

- Rutabagas

- Sprouts

- Spinach

- Watercress

---Fruits---

- Avocado

- Banana

- Coconut

- Grapefruit

- Lemon

- Tomato

- Watermelon

---Nuts---

- Almonds

- Pumpkin

- Sunflower

- Sesame

---Fats & Oils---

- Avocado

- Borage

- Evening Primrose

- Flax

- Hemp

- Olive

Table 2.0 Acid Forming Foods

- Alcohol

- Aspirin & most drugs

- Asparagus

- Beans

- Brussels Sprouts

- Catsup

- Cocoa

- Coffee

- Cornstarch

- Cranberries

- Eggs

- Flour based products

- Most meats

- Milk

- Mustard

- Olives

- Pasta

- Pepper

- Sauerkraut

- Shellfish

- Soda, soft drinks

- Sugar

- Tobacco

- Vinegar

Now, just because a particular food is acid forming does not mean that you should completely eliminate it from your diet or avoid it for an extended period of time. It just means that you shouldn't over do it, and that you should only choose about 20% of your foods from the acid forming foods list. Many foods that are acid are, in fact, quite good for you with the exception of a few.

So in closing, try as hard as you can to stick to the 80/20 rule. Your health and physique will greatly improve as a result.

WHY THE ALKALINE DIET AND CANCER IS AN IDEAL SOLUTION

As a result of the epidemic of cancer that has broken out in recent years, there have been great strides made in where cancer originated, how it grows in the body and how effective alkaline diet and cancer regime has become. The definition of cancer allows the patient to have some control in the prevention and battle of cancer cells. By sticking to a primarily alkaline diet, this reduces, and actually quenches, the production of cancer and other diseases. Because of this, an alkaline diet has been found to prevent disease, while an acidic diet encourages disease and cancer to grow.

When you take the definition of cancer simply, it is 'a malformed cell.' This malformed cell can only reproduce malformed cells, and since the human body reproduces tens of thousands of cells daily, the answer is to stop that reproduction. The best defense then is a good offense, and that is what an alkaline diet does as it feeds the good cells, while choking out the disease.

The foods that are taken into the body typically come from two categories - foods that produce an acidic environment and foods that produce an alkaline environment. If you are taking a large quantity of medicines, this might cause your system to lean more towards the acidic, but it can be counteracted by consuming more alkaline-producing foods.

An alkaline diet is generally made up of alkaline-producing foods, so that the pH level is brought to a level of around 7.4. If you search online there are alkaline/acidic charts of all the foods. If you are just beginning this diet, make a copy of the chart and carry it with you when you shop or go out to eat. In general, stay away from processed foods, fast foods fried in trans fat, any food made with white sugar or white flour, and all foods with chemicals and steroids. These foods all feed cancer cells. If this is what your diet is made up of, check the alkaline food list and see what to be eating now.

Foods on that are alkaline-producing are vegetables, seeds, most fruits, brown rice and other grains, and fish. These foods can be mixed and matched to your own preference for at least 80% of your total diet, and then you add 20% of the acidic-producing foods, and the acidic foods are not all "bad". Foods on the acidic side are whole grain breads, lean meats, milk and milk products, butter and eggs, and this adds up to make an 100% alkaline diet.

To monitor your pH level once you have gotten started on an alkaline diet and cancer fighting way of eating, check any health food store for pH strips or litmus paper.

There will be a color chart included to use and determine what your pH blood level is. For an alkaline system, it should register between 7.2 - 7.8. No two people are alike, so test your pH level about once a day as you get started. Then continue to check once a week. If you need to raise your pH level, eat more alkaline foods and use green supplements. An alkaline diet will prevent disease naturally.

THE ALKALINE DIET - WHAT CAN I EAT ON IT□

The Alkaline Diet is also known as the Alkaline Ash Diet, Alkaline Acid Diet, or the Acid Alkaline Diet.

Generally, the diet consists of eating certain citrus, other low sugar

fruits, vegetables, tubers, nuts, and legumes.

Grains, dairy products, meat, sugar, alcohol, caffeine, and fungi like mushrooms are to be avoided. By consuming such a diet, it is said that the body maintains a pH of between 7.35 and 7.45 (7.00 is neutral on the pH scale while below 7.00 is acidic).

Diet And Disease

There is some evidence that such a diet is beneficial in preventing osteoporosis and other bone health issues. However, evidence is not strong in supporting the claims that an alkaline diet may prevent or help alleviate conditions such as cancer, fatigue, obesity, or allergies.

There is, however, some evidence that cancer cells grow more quickly in an acidic environment in a laboratory setting. Therefore, a person with a predisposition to or who actually suffers from this disease may want to investigate the effects an alkaline diet have on the body.

Considering the overwhelming rise in many of these types of diseases it is easy to wonder if they are caused by the general condition of a person's internal body environment.

A wider and more scientifically vigorous examination of the Alkaline Diet is in order. However, such scientific scrutiny may be tainted from the beginning by prejudice fomented in a pharmaceutical based health care delivery system.

The theory behind the Alkaline Diet is not widely accepted by the medical community which may be one of the reasons cancer, diabetes,

and any number of other terrible diseases are at epidemic levels. The Alkaline Diet, when combined with a physically active, low stress lifestyle certainly deserves more attention from the scientific community if they can keep their bias at bay.

Diet And Disease

It would be relatively simple to see if specific conditions such as blood sugar, blood pressure, cholesterol count, and a person's weight normalize when (and if) their blood pH falls into the desired range. These symptoms occur together so often that the medical community has begun calling it Syndrome X.

If this syndrome is so common, and the protocol for scientific examination so simple, why is the Alkaline Diet still such as mystery as to whether it is beneficial or not?

It may be because there is no money to be made from recommending a specific diet.

Pharmaceutical companies test new drugs because there is a profit to be made if the drug makes it to market. But there is no profit in dietary recommendations therefore such research would fall to the universities and governmental agencies to conduct.

The fact that most of those researchers also work as consultants for the pharmaceutical industry may easily taint their enthusiasm and findings.

Good Healthy Food

So, what are you supposed to eat?

It is recommended that you avoid "acidic" foods such as sugar, red meat, shellfish, eggs, dairy, processed and other refined foods, most grains including refined grains, artificial sweeteners, alcohol, caffeine, chocolate, and soda pop.

You should consume raw fruits and vegetables that have a high chlorophyll content such as green leafy vegetables.

The brassica family of vegetables (also known as

crucifers) are well represented on the Alkaline Diet and include:

- Broccoli

- Brussels sprouts

- Cabbage

- Cauliflower

- Turnips

- Collard greens

- Kale

- Kohlrabi

- Bok Choi

- Mustard Greens

Other raw vegetables to try on your alkaline diet are:

- Avocado

- Tomato

- Red Beets

- Carrots

- Lima Beans

- Red and black radishes

- Rutabaga

- Egg plant

- Asparagus

- Artichoke

- Lettuce

- Endive

- Cucumber

- Celery

- Peppers

- Zucchini

- Squash

- Spinach

- Parsnips

- Onions

Healthy Fruit

The best fruit to consume on the alkaline diet includes:

➢ Unripe bananas

➢ Sour cherries

- ➢ Fresh coconut

- ➢ Figs (either raw or dried)

- ➢ Fresh lemon

- ➢ Lime

Whether the Alkaline Diet is as good for preventing disease as its proponents claim will have to wait to be seen.

However, following the alkaline diet certainly will keep you within the parameters of what most other medical practitioners and organizations have been claiming to be a healthy diet for many, many years.

ALKALINE FRUIT JUICES

Find Out Why Alkaline Fruit Juices Should Become A Major Part Of Your Diet

It is suggested that roughly 80 percent of our dietary intake should consist of fruits and vegetables. Drinking fruit juices will provide a great percentage of that amount. Learn which fruit drinks are included in the alkaline family.

Apples, when eaten, are a great source of vitamins and minerals. When consuming apple juice, you are getting the nutrients needed to help keep you healthy. "An apple a day..." comes to mind when thinking of the apple. Just because you may eat apples on a regular basis, you can still enjoy the flavor and benefits of drinking apple juice. Apples are rich in vitamins A, C and some B vitamins. Vitamin A is good for overall health, vitamin C helps boost the immune system, and many of the B vitamins provide energy.

Bananas are another good source of vital nutrients and vitamins. Bananas contain high levels of calcium and potassium. Calcium is great for bone development and overall good bone health. Potassium helps muscles to stay nourished. A shortage of potassium in your body could result in cramps. It is suggested that you consume a juice which contains banana. (ie. orange/banana, orange/strawberry/banana...)

Sweet grapes are another good source of alkaline juice. Any variety of sweet grapes will do. These tiny fruits contain high amounts of antioxidants and are very tasty. Most grape juices have little or no additives so they are basically pure fruit juice. Grapes contain resveratrol which keeps heart muscle flexible. It is also believed that resveratrol may reduce the risk of Alzheimer disease. Pterostilbene is an antioxidant found in grapes that helps lower cholesterol and is good for anyone who is at risk for high cholesterol.

Everyone's favorite fuzzy fruit, the peach, is another great alkaline juice fruit. Peaches and peach juice helps maintain healthy skin, hair and

nails. Peaches contain vitamin A for overall health, potassium for healthy muscles, vitamin C to help the immune system, Iron to enrich blood cells, and vitamins B-1 and B-2 which will help with energy levels. Peaches also include niacin, sodium, and phosphorus.

The best alkaline fruit juice is also the most uncommon. Fig juice tops the list when it comes to alkaline fruit juices. Fig juice is commonly used as a laxative and, therefore, rarely considered to be a drink of enjoyment. Fig juice is extremely high in vitamin B-6. It is estimated that there are 110mg of vitamin B-6 per 100g of juice.

As we can see, alkaline fruit juices have many positive ingredients necessary for good health. One key identifying factor of alkaline fruits and their juices is that they are sweet. The juices in these fruits are rarely tangy or tart like most citrus fruits. Those fruits are high in vitamin C and contain a different pH level than the alkaline fruits and juices. Regardless of the one you choose as your favorite, any and all of these fruit juices will provide a high percentage of your daily fruit intake.

THE BENEFITS OF ALKALINIZING AND MINERALIZING WATER

Kevin: Let's talk a little bit about alkalinizing water and there are a lot of machines that do that. What are the benefits of that? Do they actually take out some of the mineral content, as well? Are their filters built into some of these things or are they just changing the pH balance of the water?

Mike: Well, how these units actually work and based on just straight chemistry they produce two outputs. One output is more alkaline and the other output, the other stream of water coming out is more acidic, because you can't really change the pH of that. Let's say a pot of water you can't change the pH really, unless you add something to take something out. You would need to perform some kind of chemistry. You can split it apart. You can have one batch that's more alkaline and another batch that's more acidic. I owned a unit like that for a while and I have some very high end pH testing equipment that I use for my gardening, because if you're going to grow blueberries then you need the right pH for the soil.

Well, these units, sure they produce a little slightly more alkaline water, but it's not that big of a deal. It's really not that drastic. I found that you can create more alkaline water by stirring up some barley grass juice in a glass of water. That's far more alkaline. So if you want to drink alkaline water that's fine, but there are other ways to get that. Celery juice is very alkaline. So is cucumber juice and that's a great way to get that. The other thing people don't realize is there's a risk and a drawback to using this and that is that most people when they eat food they don't have sufficient stomach acid to properly digest that food, especially the minerals. If you want to digest calcium and magnesium and all of these minerals you need a really strong stomach acid. That's the only way you're going to break it down. Well, what if you take your mineral supplements and then you drink all this alkaline water? The fact is you're not going to be able to break down those minerals and they're going to go right for you and your going to waste your money. You might actually contribute to kidney stones or something.

There are times in your diet when you need more acid. Like when you're eating minerals, or if you eat meat for example, which I would never do, but some people do. If you eat a steak you want an acidic stomach, believe me, because you've got to break that stuff down. Dogs have very, very acidic stomachs, because they eat raw bones and they can just digest those bones with their stomach acid, but if you fed a dog alkaline water and then fed him some raw bones that dog would have some serious digestive problems. Finally, I know I'm answering this with a very long paragraph here.

Kevin: No. Keep going.

Mike: But finally, the main reason most people are drinking this alkaline water in the first place is because their regular diets or to acidic to begin with. They're using this machine as a way to compensate for really lousy dietary choices that are too acidic. So they think oh, gee, I'm going to drink a Coke and I'm going to drink a Starbucks and I'm going to have the sugar in my diet means and these are all acidic, so I'm I'm going to compensate with an alkaline water and that's the wrong approach. The right approach is just get those acidic substances out of your diet, drink some fresh water, drink some celery juice, drink some fruit juice and you're going to be fine. So personally, I don't recommend the alkaline machine. I don't see that they have important use in a healthy lifestyle, frankly.

Kevin: Yeah.

Mike: There's a lot of commercial hype out there and granted, there are some products are really great, like these water filters that are really fantastic and I mentioned I like the Aqua Sonic company. Their products really do work. Even the Pur filters and Brita filters. They really work and they take stuff out of the water and that's great, but plop down

$600 or $900 on alkalinizing machine when your stomach acid might really need to be more acidic doesn't take any sense to me.

Kevin: Yeah. I don't know what your extent of knowledge about this is,

but are we alkaline phobic? Is that the right word?

Mike: You mean are we afraid of being to alkaline?

Kevin: No. I guess that would be the wrong word, but I think we fear -

- are we acidi-phobic. I like that. Mike: Okay.

Kevin: Acidiphobic. I think of the natural health world, we might have become that a little bit.

Mike: Sure. There's a lot of legitimate research based on the idea that people are too acidic in terms of what they take in, because it's all processed foods and caffeine and sugar and phosphoric acid, which you can either drink a Coke or you can scrub anchors on battleships with it. It's a multiple purpose acid. So that's very true, but the answer, like I mentioned is not to counter that with alkaline substances, per se, but rather to remove these dangerous acids from your diet and then just eat fresh produce and drink fresh vegetable juice and eat like a freshitarian, to use that term that we talked about before. Get this, some people who have bone health problems, especially elderly people, will swallow Tums. Tums are made of some really low-grade minerals, like calcium carbonate, for example and sodium bicarbonate, which is an alkaline mineral. So they're taking calcium minerals and alkaline minerals together. What does that mean? It means that they're probably not going to be able to digest the calcium. If you were going to take calcium and you want to be able to use it you should take it with some vinegar. Drink some vinegar and take some calcium and then you get it. Think about this. Pregnant women, when they get weird cravings they sometimes make a lot of sense. One night an expectant mother can wake up and just say I want pickles and ice cream. What is pickles and ice cream? Pickles are acidic. Ice cream is calcium. It has a lot of calcium in it. She's craving calcium and her body is giving her the signal that says eat some calcium and break it down with acids and absorb it and that's why she's craving pickles and ice cream.

Kevin: It sounds awful.

Mike: Yeah, it does, but if you need calcium so desperately your body can come up with that signal.

Kevin: Right.

Mike: A lot of times during pregnancy that's exactly what's going on.

Kevin: It goes for or whatever it has recognized as the source of that?

Mike: Absolutely. Like magnesium and chocolate. People who have this craving for chocolate, often they just need more magnesium.

Kevin: Yeah.

Mike: I find that, for example, if I have a craving for salty fat foods it means I'm deficient of salt and I hope we get a chance to talk about salt and water, by the way.

Kevin: What an incredible way to move on... Let's talk about that, because the conception or misconception or the myth, which I believe it is and I just want to put that on line is that we should drink eight glasses of water a day, eight ounces and that's sufficient for everyone.

Mike: Yeah, okay. Where do we begin on this one? Well, clearly water is important to health and I'm a big advocate of drinking water, so let me put that out there first. It's not just what you drink. It's not the water that passes through your body that's important. It's the water that's hydrating your cells and your tissues and your brain. Your brain has a lot of water in it. So how do you retain this water? How you actually keep yourself hydrated at a cellular level? The answer to that is, of course, salt. You've got to have salt and I don't mean that processed sodium chloride garbage that people have too much of. I'm talking about full spectrum sea salt and Celtic sea salt. You know the rough stuff, the brown looking stuff. It's not white. It's not processed. It's full spectrum sea salt. When you get that into your body it allows you to retain the water and makes you healthy, so that you can lubricate your neurons, so that your cells can get rid of toxic byproducts that are water-soluble, so that you can circulate the vitamins and minerals that your cells need

in order to live. This water is crucial for that, but you got to have salt to keep in. You know, some people will say well, I don't want to retain water, because it makes me look fat and I noticed that, too, like when I go to the ocean and I swim in the ocean for three or four days. I get so much salt in my body that I do kind of puff up a little bit. I think last time I was there I gained 5 pounds of water weight.

Kevin: Wow.

Mike: I don't care. I'm not competing in Mr. Natural Bodybuilding contest. I'm here to be healthy and not to lose so much salt that I look ripped all the time. I want to be healthy and if I have a little bit of puffiness I know that that's associated with good hydration. The truth is I've been in cases where I exercised too much and I sweat too much, because I live in the desert and I'll run and I'll exercise and sweat out all the minerals and I'll look really thin and really fit, like a triathlete and I find I'm salt deficient. I'm craving salty snack foods. One time I found myself at Trader Joe's sleepwalking on pharmaceuticals or something, even though I don't take them, sleepwalking towards the bag of Cheetos or something. I was like, oh my gosh, what am I doing?

Kevin: Right.

Mike: Clearly I needed salt. Kevin: That's an incredible point.

THE BENEFITS OF DRINKING ALKALINE WATER

Having been a performer for the better part of my life keeping up the same energy levels on stage isn't always easy. About five years ago the signs of a volatile lifestyle were starting to really take their toll. It wasn't too long before taking extra curricular substances became a permanent fixture of every performance. I knew full well that something had to dramatically change before my health deteriorated any further. I started to juice every morning and this helped immensely but every time I did a show I still felt fatigued and depleted at the end of the night. I also noticed something else that was very strange at the time. I have always been a firm believer that consuming lots of water especially when you are perspiring so rapidly is essential in replenishing lost fluids. But for some reason even though I would drink a minimum of 2 litres a show I always felt that the bottled water I was consuming wasn't quite right. I would also feel a lot of acid reflux after the show and all through to the next morning.

So I started to diligently research alkaline water otherwise referred to as 'ionized water' and found out very quickly that the benefits from drinking it were nothing short of amazing. There was a multitude of testimonials from people all over the world attesting to its healing powers. So what is alkaline water and why is it so good for us? According to my research I found that alkaline water was able to neutralize the acidity build up in the body caused mainly by stress, modern diet, pollution in the air and even by certain brands of bottled water. The PH level of our blood fluctuates between 7.35 - 7.45 which on a PH scale is slightly alkaline. If the blood was to deviate even slightly from this figure we could potentially die.

Acidity build up in the body also creates the appropriate environment for many types of disease to flourish and expand. Scientists have found that cancer cells and tumors feed on acidity and are able to proliferate in an acidic environment. By drinking alkaline water on a daily basis you are neutralizing the acidity and free radicals in your body that we are bombarded with on a regular basis. This whole concept made a lot of sense to me and I decided to venture out and purchase myself a good

quality alkaline filter. There seem to be a lot of choices on the market but abiding by the rules of 'you get what you pay for' I decided to spend that little bit extra and get myself a reputable and good quality unit.

The Benefits

I will never forget the first time I tasted alkaline water. Unless you have tried it for yourself my description would hardly do it justice. The very first thing I noticed was how easy and smooth it was to drink. It almost has a velvet kind of consistency compared to the harshness of normal tap water. I did some further investigating and found out that 'ionization' which is the process for making alkaline water breaks clusters of water molecules into smaller micro-clusters. This greatly reduces the size of the clusters from the 11-16 molecules in standard water to just 5-6 molecules in ionized water. Smaller clusters pass through cell walls more easily and hydrate the cells more quickly. This explained why it went down so much easier than normal drinking water. It wasn't very long before I started to notice significant differences in my health and energy levels. This was no less evident on stage and the difference that it made to my performances. My energy levels were gradually improving and the need to take pharmaceutical substances for every show was a thing of the past. What's interesting is that due to the size, micro-clusters of ionized water molecules are expelled from the cells more efficiently, carrying damaging toxins out of the cells and flushing them out of the system. A higher pH level in the body also reduces the need for fat and cholesterol to protect the body from damaging acids. One of the leading causes of obesity is due to the body being forced to produce an unhealthy amount of fat cells just to stop the acidity from burning holes inside of you.

I also started to notice that cooking with alkaline water

improved the taste of foods and I found that it also enhanced the taste of various herbal teas. Cooking with normal water only adds more acidity to your diet and not to mentioned all of the other unfiltered microbes that you might be digesting. By the way boiling the water does not kill all bacteria nor does it get rid of fluoride.

My mother who has been a rheumatoid sufferer for the last 20 years also started drinking the alkaline water and noticed a dramatic change in her mobility. Normally she couldn't even get out of bed in the morning due to the excruciating pain that she felt. Any sort of arthritis is due to a build up of acidity in the joints and drinking alkaline water has helped my mother better manage this disease and the pain associated with it.

Having the alkalizing filter also prompted me to test the PH level of bottled water on the market. The results were not only surprising but at times overwhelming to say the least. Some of the bottled water that I had been drinking on a regular basis had a PH level of about 1-2 which is highly acidic. It was no wonder I consistently caught the flu and was always sick. By drinking the large amounts of this particular water I was basically created the perfect environment for pathogens and viruses to breed and flourish. There was 2 bottled brands however that did test neutral on the PH scale and if you are out and about and don't have access to alkaline water they would more than suffice. The 2 bottled brands are 'Evian' and

'Fiji Water'. They both tested between 7-8 on the pH scale which is still slightly alkaline and much healthier to consume.

INTRODUCTION TO ANTI INFLAMMATORY DIET

To discover how to regain control of your diet, it is important to understand the common thread amongst nearly all chronic disease processes known as silent inflammation. This phenomenon made big news several years ago when it was featured on the cover of the February 2004 issue of Time Magazine. It has been the subject, directly or indirectly, of thousands of scientific articles in some of the most prestigious scientific journals in the world. The vast majority of the research is pointing towards silent inflammation as the cause of diseases ranging from heart disease to Alzheimer's to many types of cancer. We will touch on the causes of silent inflammation, its impacts, and what you can do to reverse it before it's too late. The best resource to understand silent inflammation and how to reverse it is The Anti-Inflammation Zone, by Dr. Barry Sears. This book was written for the public, not for doctors, and will give you knowledge of the topic that exceeds many physicians!

Two of the major essential fatty acids in the body are omega-6 fats and omega-3 fats. Omega-3 fatty acids are found primarily in cold water fish and grass-fed meats, while grains and seed oils, such as corn oil, soybean oil, and safflower oil are rich sources of omega-6 fatty acids. Research indicates that our bodies are designed to optimally function with a ratio of omega-3 to omega-6 somewhere in the neighborhood of 1:1 to 1:4. This means for every milligram of omega-3 fat you eat, you should eat one to four milligrams of omega-6 fats. Unfortunately, the average American diet has an omega-3 to omega-6 ratio of around 1:25!

How does this cause silent inflammation? Your immune system causes any inflammation, whether acute, in the case of a sprained ankle swelling, or silent. Molecules called eicosanoids are like the generals of the immune system. Pro-inflammatory eicosanoids coordinate the bodies' response to injury, resulting in inflammation. They control molecules called macrophages, that gobble up invading tissue as well as molecules called cytokines that signal for more immune cells to move to a specific area. During the inflammatory phase of an injury, these

molecules cause the tissue to become swollen and painful. This is the bodies' way of guarding against further injury to the area, such as keeping you from placing pressure on a sprained ankle. In the case of acute inflammation, this is a wonderful, albeit sometimes painful process to speed the healing of an injury and repair the tissue.

Eventually, however, the repair and remodeling of the area is completed, and anti-inflammatory eicosanoids take over. These signal the body to halt the inflammatory response, and cause the body to proceed to the next phase of the healing process. To stay healthy, your body must maintain balance between pro and anti-inflammatory eicosanoids. If the balance is upset with too many pro-inflammatory molecules silent inflammation sets in, causing a host of health problems.

The traditional medical path for dealing with inflammation is one you are probably already familiar with. Anti-inflammatory drugs, such as aspirin, Advil, Alleve, or Tylenol cause the body to stop the production of the pain-causing eicosanoids. Unfortunately, these medications do not distinguish between the pro and anti-inflammatory eicosanoids, but decrease both. This leads to problems in the immune system ranging from stomach ulcers to even death. Over 20,0000 people a year in the United States die from the recommended use of anti-inflammatory drugs! Clearly, medications are not a good long-term solution for stopping silent inflammation.

If you wrapped a rubber band tightly around your finger, you would experience immediate throbbing pain, swelling, and eventually might even lose circulation in the finger. Medications exist that are strong enough to block the pain, but wouldn't removing the rubber band that is causing the problem in the first place be a wiser solution? By eliminating or at least drastically reducing the causes of chronic inflammation in your diet you are able to live longer, feel better, and look younger without drugs or surgery! Does this sound too good to be true? It's not!

As mentioned before, omega-6 and omega-3 fatty acids both are building blocks of eicosanoid production. However, it is crucial to remember that omega-6 fats lead to pro-inflammatory eicosanoids while

omega-3 fats are the precursors to powerful anti-inflammatory eicosanoids. The imbalance of omega-6 to omega-3 fats in the typical American diet has led to flawed immune systems that are causing silent inflammation. We are literally eating ourselves to death!

Virtually all chronic disease processes are now thought to be in some way due to silent inflammation. For years doctors have thought heart disease was merely a problem of fat from the diet clogging the arteries, causing heart disease. The plague that builds up in the arteries is rich with cholesterol, so it was believed that high cholesterol lead to heart attacks by choking off blood to the heart. The trouble with this theory is that 50 percent of all heart attacks occur in people with normal cholesterol. Another problem with this model is that as Americans steadily reduced their cholesterol intake throughout the twentieth century, heart disease not only did not decrease, it became much more prevalent!

Type II diabetes is another disease epidemic that is

rooted in silent inflammation. At its most basic level this disease, also known as non- insulin dependent diabetes mellitus (NIDDM), is caused when your cells become less responsive to the actions of the hormone insulin. Insulin is produced in the pancreas and helps glucose from the blood make its way into the cells. It is an anabolic hormone, meaning it promotes the buildup of tissue, most notably fat. So when the cells become insulin resistant and the body produces more insulin, more fat is stored. So what causes cells to become resistant to the effects of insulin? The best current research indicates that silent inflammation causes damage to the specific cells that insulin acts on to allow glucose into the cells. A study done at Louisiana State University showed that giving anti- inflammatory eicosanoids to overweight patients decreased insulin resistance by 70 percent!

After spending over $30 billion dollars on the war on cancer, our government still has not found any reliable way to prevent the disease from occurring in the first place. Any form of cancer occurs when cells in the body mutate, causing them to rapidly divide and spread. As you have learned, silent inflammation increases insulin levels in the body, which act as a fuel to spread cancer cells. This process is known as

metastasis, and it is also aided by pro-inflammatory eicosanoids found in the typical American diet.

WHAT IS INFLAMMATION IN THE BODY

A crucial question of modern life is "what is inflammation in the body" and what you can do about it. Because the crucial response is "what are you going to do about it?"

It's no secret that inflammation is the common denominator is disease today. Doctors agree it's an underlying reason for heart disease, rheumatoid arthritis and a host of other diseases.

But here's what you need to know about inflammation. It's not all bad. When you cut your finger or break a bone the swelling, redness and pain is all part of your body healing itself. And those are signs of inflammation.

The problem is when the inflammation is chronic. It's inside your body and won't stop. This is your brain sending the wrong signals to your body. Maybe you see it it terms of your throbbing wrist when the weather turns. Or, maybe you don't even know about the inflammation but it's creating all the conditions for heart disease.

Basically, chronic inflammation is your body's immune system turned on itself. It's over worked, doesn't know when to stop and the result is a serious disease. Your body attacks healthy cells and destroys them.

Here's an example of healthy inflammation, let's say you cut your finger while chopping vegetables for dinner. Your platelets rush in and a chemical cascade starts resulting in a stringy substance called fibrin. This fibrin mixes with the platelets and creates a mesh that stops the blood. It still hurts and swells and is red for a day or two but then it's fine. Doesn't even leave a scar most likely.

But let's look closer.

See, when the platelets and red blood cells rushed in, they destroyed the damaged tissue right around your cut. That prevents infection from setting in. In the process, some healthy tissue gets damaged too. That's

just part of the process. The problem is when your body doesn't know when to stop destroying tissues and just keeps going along.

Now, consider this. According to doctors, internal inflammation could cause pain from severe cramps to internal organ damage.

The scary thing is, you may very well not even know it's occurring. Most of us are at risk for chronic inflammation. It's the "Silent Killer" of the 21st century.

If you're overweight, eat a lot processed foods and don't sleep enough you could be at risk. I know, covers most of us doesn't it?

But there is something you can do about it. Getting

enough exercise and eating healthy foods are part of it. Part of your healthy diet should include plenty of omega 3 fatty acids. You can get these by eating more fish. A lot of doctors recommend fish oil supplements because they're high in omega 3's.

Omega 3's are important because they're a natural anti inflammatory.

INFLAMMATION, DISEASE AND AGING

When we think of inflammation we might think of pain and the inflammatory conditions like arthritis or gout. However, inflammation and the destruction it causes can be silent, painless and go un-noticed. Inflammation is so widely linked to heart disease, diabetes, cancer and accelerated aging. The idea that you can take a statin drug to lower cholesterol and you will somehow be protected from heart problems is for too simplified, and in a lot of respects statin drugs cause as many problems as it is supposed to solve.

Inflammation and higher levels of homeocysteine have also been linked to heart disease. Homeocysteine level is a more accurate and more important indicator to pending heart disease but is of little use to the establishment as homeocysteine levels can be reduced to safe levels with adequate amounts of the B vitamins!

Another very important fact that is well established now is for some time now, that heart disease and heart attacks rarely happen simply due to deposits of fatty plaques in our arteries. Sure arteries are active collaborators in the progress of heart disease, attracting and sheltering cells that release inflammatory substances. According to Penny Kris- Etherton, PhD, R.D, distinguished professor of nutrition at Penn State, "inflammation plays a key role in weakening arterial plaque, causing the deposits to rupture-which can lead to sudden coronary death, heart attack or stroke." These findings have also been researched and reported over the years by many.

Inflammation is not implicated just in heart disease but in all sorts of chronic diseases. So anything we do to reduce inflammation, will lower our risk of heart disease, diabetes, cancer, arthritis, asthma, speed up the aging process and so much more.

The very good news is that the amount of inflammation your body produces is within your power to control. It is entirely up to you - encourage the production of inflammation within your own body or reduce it. You choose. Interestingly prostaglandins - hormone like substances come in three main categories prostaglandins 1, prostaglandins 2, and prostaglandins 3, their main job is to increase inflammation or reduce inflammation. When, as most people do eat refined processed oils, margarine, and shortenings, causing an imbalance in the type of prostaglandins produced and ultimately this means inflammation and pain.

There are two classes of essential fatty acids we need in our diets, omega-3 and omega-6. Omega 6 is converted into two types of hormones-like substances. One type has an anti-inflammatory effect called series-1 prostaglandins, then the second type is involved in inflammation and thickening the blood called series-2 prostaglandins. The other type is series-3 prostaglandins, they have an anti- inflammatory effect. These three need to be in balance. These days the balance is tipped in favor of inflammation. We eat too many processed oils/fats, too much saturated animal fats, too much sugar and far too little in the way of fish, wild game, raw nuts and seeds or plants rich in essential fatty acids.

If we don't eat fish or wild game, which provides EPA (eicosapentaenoic acid), we do have a mechanism in place that will convert alpha-linolenic acid into EPA. However, to enable the body to convert alpha-linolenic acid to EPA, it is reliant on enough nutrients like vitamin B6, vitamin C, magnesium, and zinc. Most people on a typical diet do not get enough of these nutrients. This conversion can also be blocked by an excess consumption of processed oils, margarine and shortenings. Fruit, vegetables, nuts, seeds and whole grains are rich in Vitamins C and B6, magnesium and zinc the very nutrients needed for the conversion.

Inflammatory conditions are common these days. Is it any wonder? Our diets are blocking our natural pathways for the production of the correct amounts of series-1 and series-3 prostaglandins that help to balance inflammatory processes and disease. The amount and type of prostaglandin your body produces is directly and indirectly affected by what you eat and drink.

Foods that encourage inflammation, you have guessed it - refined

carbohydrates like the white flour products, sugar, saturated fats and

trans-fatty acids. Then meat, poultry, eggs and shellfish are all high in arachidonic acid, a compound that contributes to inflammation. This doesn't mean you shouldn't eat animal products but it does mean you should cut down and not eat too much.

Other foods associated with encouraging inflammation are wheat and many other grains, like rye, and barley, contain a protein called gluten that has been associated with inflammation. Potatoes, tomatoes, eggplants and peppers are members of the nightshade family and contain a compound called solanine that can trigger inflammation in many people, especially in arthritic types of conditions.

There is plenty of good news is nature has provided a lot of anti- inflammatory foods that decrease the body's production of inflammatory compounds, that also fight harmful free-radicals (also known to speed up the aging process). Wild-caught salmon is high in omega-3 fatty acids, which reduces inflammation (found in supermarkets in cans). Herring, mackerel and sardines are also rich in omega-3s. Take fish oil capsules especially if you eat little oily fatty fish. Other source of omega- 3s - walnuts counteract some of the inflammatory processes that lead to heart disease. They are also packed with other healthful compounds. Onions are high in quercetin, a type of antioxidant that inhibits enzymes that trigger inflammation. Other good sources of quercetin include apples, broccoli, red wine, or the red grapes. Blueberries are loaded with anthocyanins, a type of polyphenol antioxidant that boosts immunity and protects the body from free-radical damage, which triggers inflammation. Other good sources of poly-phenols include blackberries, strawberries, raspberries and cranberries. Now available in Panama but can be taken in capsule form.

Sweet potatoes or pumpkins are rich in carotenoids, antioxidants that, like anthocyanins, boost immunity and minimize inflammation. Other good sources of carotenoids are any deep orange, red, yellow and green fruits and vegetables, such as carrots, winter squash, mangoes and papayas. Dark green leaves of lettuces or herbs like parsley also do the same job. Garlic like onion is rich in sulfur compounds that stimulate the immune system by boosting the activity of natural killer and T helper cells, which manage the immune system. Garlic is also a potent anti-

inflammatory agent. Bromelain found in the pineapple stems, is an enzyme that decreases inflammation and has some immune-enhancing effects. This can be taken as a supplement.

Fresh ginger root acts as an anti-inflammatory by inhibiting COX-2 enzymes, part of the chemical pathway that produces inflammatory chemicals. Fresh ginger is easy to find in Panama. Turmeric is a spice that is important to Indian cooking, used in a lot of curries. Vitamin C is a very affective anti-inflammatory (the 5-a-day policy is a minimum every day).

INFLAMMATION AND DISEASE

There is a process in the body that is now believed by medical experts to be involved in all known disease processes from heart disease to cancer to Alzheimer's disease - inflammation. Most of you will have experienced inflammation before. Have you ever got a splinter in your finger? It got red and swollen, it may have bled a little and it was certainly hot and painful - all the classic signs of inflammation. Now, inflammation is actually a normal response to an injury like this and it serves us well. It helps to kill bacteria, parasites and viruses that try to invade us and this inflammation keeps us healthy. This type of inflammation usually demonstrates a 100 fold increase in immune system markers, such as white blood cells and cytokines like IL-6, TNF alpha, or C reactive protein (CRP).

However there is another, darker inflammatory response that happens in the body - what Dr Barry Sears calls "Silent Inflammation". This type of inflammation doesn't elicit the pain, swelling, redness and heat associated with classic inflammation and may only demonstrate a 4-5 fold increase in immune system markers - so can often be hard to detect. It can take years or even decades to develop and slowly but surely damages DNA and leads to disease. Unfortunately modern medicine is not very good at treating this type of silent inflammation. It is the result of poor lifestyle choices and changing lifestyle and nutrition is a much better tactic than using anti-inflammatory drugs.

The causes of silent inflammation are multi factorial:

- Over nutrition

- Excess alcohol

- Poor diet

- Inactivity

- Pollution

- Poor sleep

- Stress / depression

- Drug use

One of the primary sources of silent inflammation in the body is excess body fat. Fat is not just an unsightly inert substance that sits on your love handles or muffin top. It does not just serve as a reservoir of energy to be called upon when needed for energy. Fat is metabolic tissue that can cause all manner of things to happen in your body. Fat cells become infiltrated with high levels of immune cells that release inflammatory chemicals disrupting the uptake of sugar and burning of fat in liver cells contributing to insulin resistance, the onset of type 2 diabetes and narrowing arteries. Fat cells release chemicals that clot your blood, increase your blood pressure and convert inactive stress hormones into active stress hormones and contribute to conditions such as hypertension, stroke, cardiovascular disease and PCOS.

(Take home point - lose body fat)

Here is a short inflammation questionnaire developed by Dr

Barry Sears

1. Are you overweight?

2. Are you taking cholesterol medication?

3. Are you taking blood pressure medications?

4. Do you wake feeling groggy each day?

5. Do you get carbohydrate cravings?

6. Do you suffer from fatigue?

7. Dou you have brittle nails?

If you answered YES to 3 or more questions you are likely suffering from Silent Inflammation. In the following blog posts this weak I'm going to discus inflammation as the course for heart attacks (not cholesterol), inflammation and blood pressure, inflammation and cancer and inflammation and diabetes. I'll also discuss how to reduce inflammation through good nutrition, Stay posted.

Inflammation and heart disease

Now, this might be a little out there for some of you, especially as we have been brain washed in to thinking that saturated fat and cholesterol blocks arteries and causes heart attacks. But what researchers are now

finding out is that inflammation is perhaps the major player here, not cholesterol.

As I mentioned the inflammatory response gets mobilised anytime there is damage to the body. Unfortunately the body is under constant low level oxidative damage all the time from free radicals. These free radicals are nasty little unstable molecules that fly around stealing electrons from cells and generally causing havoc. The body's defence to these free radicals are antioxidants; antioxidants are able to safely donate their electrons to the free radicals rendering them safe. The main source of antioxidants in our body are formed from the food we eat, foods that contain amino acids and nutrients such as vitamin A, vitamin C, vitamin E, zinc, selenium and many other compounds such as alpha lipoic acid, green tea extract and carotenes.

The classic heart disease theory looks a little like this:

Too much cholesterol in the diet causes cholesterol to be deposited in the arteries, such as the coronary arteries.

Cholesterol deposited in the coronary arteries causes narrowing or blocked arteries and hey presto a heart attack.

A novel approach to heart disease involving inflammation looks like this:

A poor diet lacking in antioxidants leads to poor protection from free radicals and oxidative damage.

As cholesterol travels though the arteries it moves in and out of the vascular epithelial cells.

Cholesterol is attacked by free radicals and becomes damaged "oxidised

cholesterol".

Oxidised cholesterol is not recognised by the by the immune system which mounts an inflammatory reaction whereby immune cells called macrophages come along and eat the oxidised cholesterol.

The macrophage that has eaten the damaged cholesterol becomes a foam cell that is now trapped inside the epithelial cells that line the walls of the arteries.

As these foam cells build up they cause narrowing of the artery and can lead to reduced blood flow to the heart muscle.

Hey presto a heart attack.

So cholesterol just seems to be the innocent bystander of the oxidative damage caused by a diet lacking antioxidants.

Consider these couple of studies to highlight the point:

The JUPITER study in 2008 investigated 17,000 people considered not to be at risk for heart disease. This trial assessed whether the statin drug Crestor could prevent heart disease in healthy individuals with low LDL-cholesterol levels but elevated CRP (a marker for inflammation).

The study found "unequivocal evidence of a reduction in cardiovascular morbidity and mortality (about 40%) among those treated with the statin compared with placebo". However what mechanism was at work? We know that the study group had low cholesterol so was lowering it even more what helped, or do statins lower CRP and prevent heart disease by reducing inflammation.

Another study called The Lyon Diet Heart Study investigated 600 people who had survived a first heart attack and were at high risk of another. The authors divided the people in to one of two groups:

Group 1 received no dietary intervention.

Group 2 received advice to follow a Mediterranean diet (More on this later).

What were the results? Well, as with the JUPITER

trial, The Lyon Diet Heart Study was also stopped early because those following the Mediterranean diet had such a significant reduction in recurrent heart attacks that the authors were ethically compelled to put everyone on a Mediterranean diet. After 4 years, those still following a Mediterranean diet had a 50-70% lower risk of recurrent heart attacks! Compare this to the JUPITER study where those taking a drug only had a 40% reduction in cardiovascular morbidity and it's quite plain to see that making significant changes in your diet and lifestyle are far more effective for preventing heart disease than taking drugs.

The Mediterranean diet

The Mediterranean diet is generally considered to be the native diet of the inhabitants of Crete from between 1945 to 1970. It consists of the following foods:

- Abundant in plant food (fruits, vegetables, pulses, beans and lentils, whole grains, nuts and seeds)

- Fresh fruit as the typical daily dessert

- Olive oil as the principle source of fat

- Saturated fat less than 8% of total calories

- Moderate dairy products mainly cheese and yoghurt

- Moderate fish, lamb and poultry

- Low red meat

- Less than 4 eggs a week

- Moderate wine consumption 1-2 glasses a day

- Less than 2000 calories a day

- This diet may be moderate to low in saturated fat, but it is high in omega 3 fats, fibre and antioxidants that help prevent inflammation.

Inflammation and high blood pressure

Dr Barry Sears' "silent inflammation" not only contributes to heart disease but also to high blood pressure or what is sometimes referred to as hypertension. Now, hypertension is somewhat of a unique disease as there aren't any noticeable symptoms in the early stages, so it's a good idea to get your blood pressure checked and do all you can to keep it in the "normal" zone.

Many of you will have gone to the GP and had your blood pressure measured. You may have been told that you blood pressure is 120 over 80 or 135 over 90, but what do these number actually mean?

When your heart beats it forces blood out in to the arteries, which produces the first number in a BP reading. This number should be 120mmHg, which is considered normal, any higher than 140mmHg would be considered bad, conversely if that number is too low it can also

be bad. However if the arteries were not strong or did not produce some resistance against the pressure of the blood being pumped out by the heart, the arteries would rip open. This resistance produced by the arteries is the second number in a BP reading. This number should be 80mmHg, which is considered normal, any higher that 90mmHg would be considered bad, conversely if that number is too low it can also be bad.

From scientific research we can make estimations about your life expectancy based on your blood pressure, as you can see the higher your blood pressure the shorter your life expectancy.

- BP of 130/90 = 67 ½ years

- BP of 140/95 = 62 ½ years

- BP of 150/100 = 55 years

The arteries are not just static tubes thorough which the blood flows, they are able to constrict and dilate depending on different factors such as stress, smoking and nutritional status. If a tube through which a fluid is moving narrows, the pressure in that tube increases, conversely if it widens, the pressure in the tube decreases much like what happens in arteries.

Many of you will have heard that if you are overweight

or eat too much salt you will have higher blood pressure, and that to reduce blood pressure you need to reduce salt in the diet - true, but this is not the only mechanism at work here. Inflammation also plays a big role in high blood pressure.

To understand this we need to learn a little bit about vascular biology (I can see your eyes glazing over but bear with me). The arteries are lined with cells called endothelial cells that produce a host of chemicals that can constrict or dilate your arteries. One of the major vasodilators produced by endothelial cells is nitric oxide, Nitric oxide basically tells the arteries to relax and widen, which will reduce blood pressure. What we know is that C-reactive protein (CRP) that inflammatory cytokine that I mentioned earlier can decrease the production of endothelial nitric oxide and increase inflammatory nitric oxide, leading to vasoconstriction

and increased blood pressure. Inflammation basically devours nitric oxide. We also know that oxidative damage and free radicals reduces nitric oxide, and that hypertensive patients have reduced antioxidants such as glutathione, superoxide dismutase, vitamin E, vitamin C, vitamin A, copper, and polyunsaturated fats.

So there you have it - inflammation causes increased blood pressure.

One thing that has been shown to reduce blood

pressure is something called the DASH (Dietary Approaches to Stop Hypertension) diet. The DASH diet is essentially a low salt, low carb diet that is higher in protein and essential fats.

- Meat poultry and oily fish 2-4 servings a day

- Vegetables 6-8 servings a day

- Fruits 4 servings a day

- Dried beans, seeds and nuts 1-2 servings a day

- Low fat dairy products 1-2 servings a day

- Cereals, grains and pasta 1-2 servings a day

- Fats and oils 4-5 servings a day (mainly unsaturated fats like olive oil, fish oil, however some saturated fat is allowable)

- Fibre - 50g a day (mix of soluble and insoluble fibre - may need to use a fibre supplement)

Again this diet is lower in inflammatory foods and higher in antioxidants much like the Mediterranean diet I mentioned earlier (in fact there are many similarities).

Inflammation and cancer

A growing number of cancer researchers are coming to the conclusion that cancer is basically an inflammatory disease and that the longer there is inflammation present in a tissue or an organ, the higher the risk of associated carcinogenesis.

Epidemiological studies estimate that nearly 15 percent of worldwide cancers are associated with microbial infection; this may include cervical cancer and the HPV1 virus, bowel cancer and inflammatory bowel

disease due to bacterial dysbiosis and stomach cancer secondary to H. Pylori infection. All of these infectious agents are associated with an inflammatory response in the body.

One way the immune system deals with these invaders is to release free radicals that kill the invading viruses and bacteria. However, these free radicals can also damage the DNA of healthy cells. These cells either repair themselves or die. If a large number of cells in an area dies secondary to infection there is an inflammatory mediated response that may lead to tumour growth.

Many other cancers may be the result of long term chronic irritation and inflammation such as in smoking and lung cancer or chemical toxicity (xenoestrogens) and breast cancer. Once again there is DNA damage, inflammation cell death and tumour growth.

Eventually these tumours are capable of releasing inflammatory chemicals that can maintain their growth, such as by initiating the growth of new blood vessels that feed tumour growth.

I'm not going to present an "anti cancer" diet, but I am going to suggest that sugar could be a contributing cause to cancers. Cancer loves sugar is a statement that seems to get banded around. Cancer cells appear to use a combination of lots of sugar and specific proteins to ignore cellular instructions to die off and keep growing. Plus we know that people who consume more omega 3 fats, antioxidants and fibre suffer less from cancer. So by eating a diet that is anti-inflammatory such a diet rich in oily fish, fruits and vegetables may protect you from cancer.

Inflammation and diabetes

Inflammation might also be a cause for type 2 diabetes. This type of diabetes is generally considered to be the results of being overweight and from eating too much sugar which makes the cells resistant to the effects of insulin.

But what might actually be the cause is... inflammation!

I've already discussed how being overweight causes the release of a whole load of inflammatory chemicals that contribute to what Dr Barry Sears calls "silent inflammation". Well, research on mice shows that inflammation provoked by immune cells called macrophages (the same cells that become foam cells and lead to blocked arteries - and that are also concentrated in fat cells) leads to insulin resistance and type 2 diabetes.

This research was done in mice that were genetically engineered to lack a specific gene present in the insulin-producing cells of the pancreas. These genes are sensitive to the inflammatory response caused by macrophages and when these mice lacked the gene they did not develop diabetes, even when fed an extremely high-fat diet.

Now this research was done in mice and applying it to humans needs to be taken cautiously, however there is a good argument to reduce inflammation to protect the pancreas.

Other anti-inflammatory foods that can be very useful in protecting yourself from "silent inflammation" include:

- Oily fish rich in omega 3 fats

- Ginger

- Garlic

- Turmeric

- Quercitin found in onions, broccoli, tea, wine and grapes.

CONTROLLING ARTHR...
INFLAMMATION AND PA...

Most of us by now know that it is important to eat fish and to take our fish oils to keep our memory sound and our joints lubricated. However what do we do when despite our best efforts our body is beginning to seize up and we have pain in our joints and cramps and we have arthritis?

Inflammation is often directly responsible for joint pain and tissue damage in Arthritis. It is important to choose foods that decrease inflammation such as avoiding refined, processed and manufactured foods since these contain inflammatory fats, preservatives and carbohydrates.

It is possible to increase inflammation with Omega 6 fatty acids. They are found in soybean oil which is often used in biscuits and biscuit snacks. Another problem is corn syrup which is often used as sweetener. It is a carbohydrate that we digest quickly but disturbs the metabolism leading to the body making inflammation in some instances.

On the other hand extra-virgin olive oil has the antioxidant (polyphenol) which helps protect tissues from inflammation. Omega 3 (oily fish such as salmon, sardines and herring) will help reduce inflammation. We

times a week but as we all know fish
ssential for people with arthritis.

t to distinguish good carbohydrates
nding the glycemic index and how
l sugar. Controlling blood sugar
inflammation so replace high-glycemic foods
made with sugar and flour with lower type foods such as
whole grains, sweet potatoes, beans and squash. If you
must eat pasta then do so but not too often. It is better than
bread and potatoes. You also need less animal protein,
especially red meat and chicken as these contain an amino
acid which may cause inflammation. Instead eat more
vegetable protein such as beans and soy. It is also
important to check if you have wheat and yeast
sensitivities as these can add to your problems for all your
cells in your body.

Fruit and vegetables are a must on your list.
Choose three from each colour daily and add ginger
and turmeric, both which have anti- inflammatory
effects. Green tea also makes for a good anti-
inflammatory drink.

From the list of supplements which will help Celery is
essential for arthritis as it has anti-inflammatory and anti-
rheumatic properties. It is detoxifying, helps the kidneys
dispose of waste products and is good for the digestion. It
is useful with bio-flavanoids for rheumatism and gout.

Glucosamine hydrochloride is another supplement which may regenerate cartilage and synovial fluid. It is important that you take it at the same time each day and 2 capsules a day. You will not see the effects until after about 3-6 weeks and do not take it if you are allergic to seafood. Sometimes is can upset your stomach a bit and give you loose bowel motions but this only happens in a few people. It is only a temporary measure and you need to tell your doctor if you are a diabetic or are on certain medications.

Another product in the glucosamine group is Glucosamine Sulphate which is a natural constituent of our bodies formed from glucose. It is important in making cartilage and synovial fluid that helps cushion the joints. As we age our ability to make this decreases and it has been found to stop the pain of Osteoarthritis in some cases. It may also be used as a preventative. It is good for knee Osteoarthritis and sometimes better than ibuprofen. It helps athletes and sports people reduce risk of training injuries. Arthritis sufferers should take 1500mg for acute pain followed by 500-1000mg for general maintenance. It does not act as quickly as medication and should be taken at least 6 weeks.

Since everyone is different if you do not have success with the above try Devils Claw which is yet another herbal remedy to reduce inflammation and pain. Take 1-2ml of the tincture three times a day.

If you have had success with homeopathic remedies then try some Bryonia which can help in rheumatism and arthritis, chest conditions

and headaches. Get it from a homeopath. It often assists with swollen, intensely painful joints in rheumatism.

If you prefer something more in the line of teas, try some Cats Claw which is a woody vine grown in rainforests of Peru. Traditionally the Indians used it to treat Arthritis. It has immune stimulating, anti viral, antioxidant, anti- inflammatory effects and has some anti-tumour and anti-microbial properties. It also comes in capsules.

Remember also that your digestion is important as it is important to have a good digestion to actually absorb the supplements you are taking and your nutrition from your food. Otherwise you are loading up with pills and they are just going straight through you with hardly any beneficial effects. Ginger has warming properties, is good for the digestion, circulation, helps with the inflammation and lowers blood pressure. It also helps reduce the pain. Studies in Copenhagen have found it is as effective as non-steroidal anti-inflammatory drugs but without their side effects. However it is slower to work and takes about three weeks to ease symptoms. 500mg daily is a good preventative or for long-term ailments.

To add to the above there are 12 Biochemic tissue salts which help to create a balance back to the body. Ferr Phos (phosphate of iron) is used in acute attacks with fever, inflammation of joints which are swollen and red or painful when aggravated by motion. Nat Phos (sodium phosphate) is useful when there are acid conditions and alternate it with Nat Sulph (Sodium sulphate) Nat Mur (Sodium chloride - which is ordinary salt) when there is creaking of the joints, Mag Phos (magnesium phosphate) alternated with Calc Phos (calcium phosphate) for pain relief in Osteo-arthritis. Sometimes it is good to combine Ferr Phos, Nat Phos, Nat Sulph and Silica and this was a remedy called Zief developed way back in 1964 for pain. It is important to get the chewable, biochemic salts as these are usually more effective.

The above is a long list and I cannot emphasise enough that different things work well for different people however It is possible to control Arthritis with proper diet, alkalising your system and proper supplements. Consult your natural practitioner for a balanced health

plan. It is important to not 'self-medicate' so to speak and a 10 minute chat with a practitioner at a health food store does not suffice. You need a proper, in-depth assessment by a Naturopath or Nutritionist who will make a plan to specifically suit your needs and take into account other illnesses and symptoms also.

ANTI INFLAMMATORY DIET PLAN

Some of our bodies are already on fire on the inside, and some of our habits are the same as throwing petrol on that fire.

That's what I will explain today - How to put that fire out, or at least get it back under control.

Just to recap, inflammation is the body's biological response of attempting to protect itself. It aims to remove harmful stimuli, such as pathogens, damaged cells and irritants; this is the first step of the healing process.

Inflammation triggers a response from the immune system. Initially inflammation is beneficial as it is used for protection but a lot of the time inflammation can lead to further inflammation (Chronic) which leads to big health problems.

The five signs to look out for inflammation are pain, redness, heat, swelling and loss of function!

What causes the inflammation in the first place?

- Chronic infections

- Obesity

- Environmental toxins (food, water & air)

- Physiological stress

- Intensive /endurance training

- Physical trauma

- Age

- Autoimmune disease

If you notice that in the brackets for environmental toxins is food. In this article I want to discuss the anti inflammatory diet.

Every food we eat gets a response from the body.

There are certain foods contained in many people's diet today which lead to an increase in inflammation. You can probably guess what kinds of foods these are (fake foods, fried foods, processed foods, refined carbs, coffee, alcohol).

The anti inflammatory diet contains many foods, which I have recommended for other purposes which help to stop and reduce inflammation.

It is a very natural way of improving your health and recovering from

illness or injury.

Without inflammation to worry about you will be a lot healthier and less at risk of picking up some very harmful illnesses in the long run.

So what makes up the anti inflammation diet?

This diet is made up of a variety of natural foods packed with nutritional value. There are no processed foods and everything is healthy and wholesome.

So here are the main foods which are contained in the anti inflammation diet:

Inflammation Fighting Fats!

Healthy fats make up a large proportion of the anti inflammation diet. Foods high in Omega-3 fatty acids have been proven to be anti inflammatory so I recommend eating as many of these foods to help fight inflammation.

Fish is a great source so stock up on sardines, salmon, herring and anchovies. Other good sources include extra virgin olive oil, coconut oil, avocado oil and walnuts.

Antioxidant Rich Fruit and Vegetables

Fruit and vegetables are packed full of antioxidants and vitamins,some of these vitamins are proven to be anti inflammatory. Some of the best sources of vegetables include onions, spinach, sweet potato, peppers, garlic, broccoli and other green leafy vegetables.

Good fruits and berries to look out for are blueberries, papaya, pineapple and strawberries. They are packed with high antioxidant content which is great on such a diet.

High Quality Protein

Which proteins you eat are very important. There is a big difference between cheap value meats and grass fed organic meats. The cheap value meats will most likely be packed with hormones and pesticides, which lead to inflammation, whereas grass fed organic meat will help to fight inflammation.

Pick your meat wisely and go for the omega-3 packed grass fed versions as often as you can. Use this rule when it comes to eggs as well. Steak, fish, eggs and poultry and beans (legumes).

These three types of foods form the cornerstone of the anti inflammation diet.

Also herbs and spices including ginger, curcumin, turmeric, oregano and rosemary contain important substances which reduce inflammation and help to limit dangerous free radical production.

Food to Avoid at All Costs on an Anti Inflammation Diet

I have just mentioned the foods that can lead to a reduction of inflammation which will keep you healthy. These foods I'm about to mention are the foods which cause inflammation and you should really avoid these.

It's a balancing act.

Pro Inflammatory foods:

- Processed foods

- Fast food and take aways - deep fried foods especially

- Omega 6 fats - you can find these in many oils like sunflower and soybean oil.

- Bread - most wheat and gluten containing products

- All trans-fats

- Sugar and flour

- Bacon and sausages

- Margarine

Tips to Starting Your Anti Inflammation Diet

The first steps, as with a lot of good diets are to begin to cut out the foods that are holding you back.

So if you regularly eat any of the above foods just mentioned then you need to start to cut them out. Eating these types of foods on an anti inflammation diet completely defeats the purpose of what you are trying to do and will ruin your results.

Even if you don't suffer from inflammation but want to change your eating habits then following this type of diet will still be good for you. It will increase your health greatly and will help with fat loss.

The next steps would be to begin to introduce anti inflammation foods into your diet. Begin with adding the healthy omega 3 fats. Start to use extra virgin olive oil with your vegetables, coconut oil with your cooking, start snacking with nuts instead of chocolate bars and crisps and start to eat more fresh fish.

Supplementing with a high quality fish oil supplement is also very important.

Hopefully you already eat a lot of fruit and vegetables in your diet, if not then you should start to add them now.

One of the great things about fruit and veg is variety.

There are literally hundreds of different varieties of fruit and vegetables available to us, all packed with goodness and FLAVOUR.

Drink green tea - Drinking green tea is proven to have anti inflammatory benefits. Flavonoids in the tea have anti inflammatory compounds which have been shown to reduce the risk of certain illnesses and diseases. Beware that green tea contains caffeine.

Experiment with herbs and spices - Bring some life to your cooking and start to mix things up. Many people when cooking will add salt, sugar, mayonnaise and other easy options. Start to add garlic, ginger, turmeric, cayenne and other herbs and spices to give your meal some real flavour without sacrificing the healthiness of the meal.

Cut out foods that cause problems - If you find that you are intolerant to certain foods or you suffer from problems after eating certain foods then cut them out completely. Many people get bad reactions from wheat and gluten containing foods so try cutting out these foods and see if you notice a difference. Eliminate the foods that you suspect cause problems one by one and you will soon uncover the culprit!

EATING ANTI-INFLAMMATORY FOODS

Are there really diets out there that can reduce inflammation? Do they work? Scientists have found that there is a relationship, in part, between what we eat and inflammation. They've even identified some compounds in food that can reduce inflammation and others that promote it. There is still a lot to learn about just how diet and inflammation interact, and research, as of yet, is not at that point where a specific foods or groups of foods can be singled out as being beneficial for people with arthritis. We are beginning to get a clearer picture of how eating the right way can reduce inflammation.

So why are we so concerned about inflammation? Inflammation is the body's natural defense to infections and injuries. When something goes wrong the body's immune system goes to work to inflame the area, which serves to get rid of the invader or to heal the wound. Inflammation can cause pain, swelling, redness, and warmth, but this goes away as soon as the problem is solved. This is good inflammation.

Then we have chronic inflammation, the type that's familiar to people with rheumatoid arthritis (RA), lupus, psoriatic arthritis, and other types of "inflammatory" arthritis. Chronic inflammation is the type that will not go away. All the types of arthritis that are mentioned above are a disorder of the immune system creates inflammation and then doesn't know when to shut off. Inflammatory arthritis, chronic inflammation can have serious consequences, permanent disability and tissue damage can be one if it isn't treated properly. Inflammation has been linked to a full host of other medical conditions.

Inflammation has been found to contribute to atherosclerosis, which is when fat builds up on the lining of arteries, raising the risk of heart attacks. Also, high levels of inflammation proteins have been found in the blood of people with heart disease. Inflammation has also been linked to obesity, diabetes, asthma, depression, and even Alzheimer disease and cancer. Scientists think that a constant level of inflammation in the body, even if the level is low, can have a number of negative effects. Research shows that diet can reduce inflammation; in

theory an inflammation-lowering diet should have an effect on a wide range of health conditions.

Researchers have looked for clues in the eating habits of our early ancestors to discover which foods might benefit us the most. They believe those habits are more in tune to our eating habits with how the body processes and uses what we eat and drink. Our ancestor's diet consisted of wild lean meats (venison or boar) and wild plants (green leafy vegetables, fruits, nuts, and berries). There were no cereal grains until the agriculture revolution (about 10,000 years ago). There was very little dairy, and there were no processed or refined foods. Our diets are usually are high in meat, saturated (or bad) fats, and processed foods, and there is very little exercise. Nearly everything we eat is available close by or as far away as our computer and the click of a mouse.

Our diet and lifestyles are way out of whack with how our bodies are made from the inside out. While our genetic make-up has changed very little from our early beginnings, our diet and lifestyles have changed a great deal and the changes have gotten worse over the last 50 to 100 years. Our genes haven't had a chance to adapt. We aren't giving our bodies the right kind of fuel, it's as though we think of our bodies as engines in a jet plane when instead they are like the engine in the very first planes. There are some foods that we are putting into our bodies, especially because we are eating way too much of them, that are affecting our health in a bad way.

There are two nutrients in our diets that have attracted attention, are omega-3 fatty acids and omega-6 fatty acids have been part of our diets for thousands of years. They are components in just about all of our many cells and are important for normal growth and development. Both of these acids play a role in inflammation. In several studies it was found that certain sources of omega 3's in particular, help to reduce the inflammation process and that omega 6's will raise it.

Now this is the problem, the average American eats on average about

15 times more omega 6's than omega 3's. While our very early ancestor's ate omega 6's and omega 3's in equal ratio, and it is believed

that this is what helped to balance their ability to turn inflammation on and off. The imbalance of omega 3's and omega 6's in our diets is believed to contribute to the excess of inflammation in our bodies.

So why is it that we eat so many omega 6's now? Vegetable oils such as corn oil, safflower oil, sunflower oil, cottonseed oil, soybean oil, and the products made from them, such as margarine, are loaded with omega 6's. Even many of the processed snack foods that are so readily available today are full of these oils. Based on the best information of the time, was to use vegetable oils like those mentioned above instead of foods with saturated fats such as butter and lard. It looks like the consequences of that advice may have contributed to the increased consumption of omega 6's and therefore causing an imbalance of omega 3's and omega 6's.

You can find omega 6's in other common foods such as meats and egg yolks. The omega 6 found in meat is the fatty acids that come from grain-fed animals such as cows, lambs, pigs and chickens. Most of the meat sold in America is grain fed unlike their grass-fed cousins who contain less of those fatty acids. Wild game such as venison and boar are lower in omega 6's and fat and higher in omega 3's than the meat that comes from the supermarkets where we shop.

You can get omega 3s in both animal and plant food. Our bodies can convert omega 3s from animal sources into anti-inflammatory compounds more easily than the omega 3s from plant sources. Plant foods contain hundreds of other healthful compounds many of which that are anti-inflammatory, so don't discount them all together.

There are many foods that are high in omega 3s and that include fatty fish, especially fish from cold waters. Of course everyone knows about salmon but did you know that you can also find omega 3s in mackerel, anchovies, sardines, herring, striped bass, and bluefish. It's also widely known that wild fish are better sources of omega 3s than the farm raised ones. You can also buy eggs that have been enriched with omega 3 oils. There are several excellent sources of omega 3s in plants that are leafy greens (like kale, Swiss chard, and spinach) as well as flaxseed, wheat germ, walnuts, and their oils.

You can also get omega 3s in supplements (often as fish

oil); this source has been shown to be beneficial in some instances. You should take with your doctor before you take a fish oil supplement because it can interact with some medications and under certain circumstances can increase the risk of bleeding. I take a prescribed omega 3 supplement because my doctor had told me that the ones you get in the supermarket or health food store are not pure, they have other additives that do absolutely nothing to help. There are other fats that are contributors to clogged arteries, the "bad" or saturated fats found in meats and high- fat dairy foods, these are called pro-inflammatory.

There are also the Trans fats that are relatively new to the cause of heart disease. These Trans fats can be found in processed convenience and snack foods and can be spotted by reading the labels. They can be identified as partially hydrogenated oils, often soybean oil or cottonseed oil. But, they can also occur naturally in small amounts in animal foods. The thought is that they contribute to the pro-inflammatory activities in our bodies and the amounts we eat today are staggering.

Antioxidants are substances that prevent inflammation causing "free radicals" from over taking our bodies. Plant foods such as fruits, vegetables (including beans), nuts, and seeds carry high amounts of antioxidants. Extra-virgin olive oil and walnut oil are very good sources of antioxidants, also. These foods have long been considered the basics for good health, and can be found in fruits and vegetables with colorful and vibrant pigments. The more colorful the plant, the better they are for you, from green vegetables, especially leafy ones, to low-starch vegetables, such as broccoli and cauliflower, to berries, tomatoes, and brightly colored orange and yellow fruits and vegetables.

I bet you're wondering what this has to do with Arthritis. Well, there has been some research on diet and arthritis, mostly focusing on RA. There was a study that looked into a bunch of other studies on diet and RA and found that diets high in omega 3's had some effect on reducing the symptoms of RA. There was yet another study published in 2008, that found eating omega 6 fatty acids and omega 3 fatty acids in a ratio of 2 or 3 to 1 (a low ratio compared to the 15 to 1 ratio in most people's

diet) decreased the inflammation in people with RA. There was also another study that found taking omega 3 may also allow people to reduce their use of no steroidal anti-inflammatory drugs (NSAIDs), such as ibuprofen (Advil, Motrin) and naproxen (Aleve). But these and other studies don't offer enough evidence to prove that there is any particular anti-inflammatory diet that can have a real impact on arthritis symptoms. It doesn't mean that the diets are harmful; it just means that there may come a day when research may be able to prove their benefits. In the future, diet may be considered one of the many tools along with exercise and medicine that can be used to ease the symptoms of arthritis.

We don't have to revert back completely to the caveman to eat the anti- inflammatory way to benefit from the anti-inflammatory diet. Just eating a healthful diet that is recommended today is right on track. Our chief strategy should be to balance the amount of modern day foods with the foods of long ago, which were rich in the inflammation reducing foods. Really, all we have to do is replace foods rich in omega 6 with foods rich in omega 3, cutting down on how much meat and poultry we eat while eating oily fish a couple of times a week and adding more varieties of colorful fruits and vegetables, and while whole grains were not a part of our early ancestor's diet, it should be included in ours. Be sure that it is whole grains and not refined grains because they contain many beneficial nutrients and inflammation-tempering compounds. Researchers have found that eating a lot of foods high in sugar and white flour may promote inflammation, although there is more studying that needs to be done on the subject.

The amounts of knowledge we have on how the body works and how our ancestor's ate is helping to confirm the old adage: "You are what you eat." But, there is still more we need to learn before we can prescribe any one anti-inflammatory diet. Our genetic makeup and the severity of our health condition will determine the benefits we get from an anti-inflammatory diet and unfortunately there is doubt that there will be one diet that fits us all.

Also, what we eat or don't eat is just a small part of the whole story. We are not as physically active as our ancestors and physical activity has

its own anti-inflammatory effects. Our ancestors were also much leaner than we are and body fat is active tissue that can make inflammatory producing compounds.

Anti-inflammatory eating is a way of selecting foods that are more in tune with what the body actually needs. We can achieve a more balanced diet by going back to our roots. If you look at the diet of the people of the Bible, you will find that they, like our caveman ancestors, were more active and their diets consisted of much the same things as our caveman ancestors. They also had no choice but to walk everywhere they wanted to go, there was no such thing as cars or trucks. While we have it easier today, our health has suffered greatly from it.

THE IMMUNE SYSTEM, INFLAMMATION, AND CANCER

THE IMMUNE SYSTEM EXPLAINED

The immune system is wonderful system of cells and signaling cytokines that fight infections and keep us healthy. We come in contact with billions of microorganisms every day. These include bacteria, viruses, fungi, and parasites. To protect us, we have an immune system. The immune system is a fascinating collection of infection fighting white blood cells and their partners the complement system and cytokines.

The complement system contains small proteins which circulate throughout the blood system. Their job is to recognize foreign substances (antigens), bind to them, and then activate the rest of the system. They stick to the bad cells and mark them so that the other immune cells can recognize the infectious cells. Another role of the complement system is to kill bacteria.

The next group is phagocytes. These cells can eat bacteria a process called phagocytosis. The phagocytes include granulocytes, macrophages which are converted monocytes, and dendritic cells. This system of cells is the first line of defense against infections.

Lymphocytes make up the next set. There are different types of lymphocytes and each has a specific function. T-helper cells are the main regulators of the immune system. When they come in contact with an antigen presenting cell such as a macrophage that has just eaten a bacteria, the helper cell is activated and it then helps turn on the rest of the immune system. Another type of T-cell is a killer T-cell. These cells circulate in the body looking for infections or infected normal cells, or even cancer cells. Their job is quite simple, when they find a bad cell, they kill it. B-lymphocytes help the immune system kill bacteria by producing immunoglobulins. Immunoglobulins act as tags that mark bacteria for removal by the phagocytes. These are produced every time you get and infection or an immunization. When the same bug invades your body, the B-lymphocytes remember and then produce more immunoglobulins via the plasma cells to help kill the infection.

Finally, there are substances called cytokines. These substances are used for a variety of purposes. They help the cells signal to each other, they can act as growth factors, they recruit immune cells, theyactivate immune cells, they turn off immune cells, and some even act as hormones. The cytokines are very important to keep the system running and they need to be in a balance. There are cytokines to turn on the system and to turn off the

136

system. When there is an imbalance, the end result is either an immune deficiency or an overactive immune system. The overactive immune system is what is involved in chronic inflammation and this is a bad thing because of the diseases chronic inflammation causes. In fact, chronic inflammation has been implicated in heart disease, stroke, dementia, and cancer.

INFLAMMATION AND CANCER

We have known about inflammation and cancer since 1863 when Rudolph Virchow discovered white blood cells in tumor tissues. Today, the connection between chronic inflammation and cancer is commonly accepted. Some common examples of cancers resulting from chronic inflammation include ulcerative colitis and Crohn's disease leading to bowel cancers. Barrett's esophagus results in cancer of the esophagus. Celiac disease can lead to small bowel lymphomas. Hashimoto's thyroiditis can lead to lymphoma of the thyroid.

Inflammation stimulates tumor development at all stages; initiation, progression, and metastasis. Tumor initiation is the process when a normal cell becomes malignant. Tumor progression is the process by which the cancer cell grows, and metastasis is the process by which the cancer cell spreads to distant sites either through the lymphatics to the lymph nodes or through the blood to distant organs.

The role inflammation plays in tumor cell initiation is clear but the mechanism is not worked out yet. It is thought to be a two part process. The inflammatory cells are responsible for secreting reactive oxygen species (ROS) and reactive nitrogen species (RNS). These normally are used to kill bacteria or virus-infected normal cells. In a chronic state, these ROS and RNS can damage the DNA of normal cells causing

mutations. A mutation in an oncogene can be the initial process that eventually leads to a cancer. The second step is the inflammatory cells secrete cytokines that increase cell growth, so not only are the cells stimulated to grow but they are doing so in an environment full of ROS and RNS setting up a perfect situation to produce mutated oncogenes.

The manner in which chronic inflammation encourages tumor cell progression is not well described. It is thought that the inflammatory cytokines produce many effects especially growth promotion and degradation of the tissues surrounding the tumor (stromal matrix) which helps tumor cells spread and migrate.

Finally, the milieu of cytokines also encourages metastasis. Some of them serve as growth factors for blood vessel formation. This is called angiogenesis and it is necessary for tumor cells to metastasize. Additionally, as the blood vessels are being formed around the tumor cell, additional cytokines have protease activity which break down the stromal matrix and allow the cancer cells to migrate in to the blood vessel and then metastasize.

When the immune system is in good working order, we remain in the best of health protected from infections and also cancers. A healthy immune is our best defense, but what foods are best for your immune system? Here is a list, and as always, it is best to get these nutrients directly from foods rather than a pill.

NINE OF THE BEST IMMUNE BOOSTING NUTRIENTS

- Vitamin C: Increases the production of white blood cells, antibodies, and the production of interferon. Only 200 mg/day is necessary. Mega doses end up in the toilet. It is best to get your vitamin C from citrus fruits, green peppers, strawberries, tomatoes, broccoli, and sweet and white potatoes.

- Vitamin E: Improves natural killer cell and B cell function. It can be found in seeds, oils and grains.

- Carotenoids: Vitamin A and beta-carotene increase infection fighting cells and are powerful anti-oxidants. They have also been found to have anti-cancer activity and can be found in greenleafy

- vegetables, intensely colored vegetables, fish, fish, eggs, and dairy products.

- Bioflavenoids: Are anti-inflammatory and anti-viral. They improve cell walls and are essential to absorb vitamin C. Bioflavenoids can be found along side vitamin C in citrus fruits.

- Zinc: Improves production of white blood cells especially T cells. Zinc has been shown in clinical studies to duration of common cold. You can find zinc in peanuts, peas, lentils, and lima beans.

- Garlic: Boosts white blood cells, natural killer cells, and production of antibodies. It also has direct anti-bacterial effects. Try to add garlic whenever possible to your diet.

- Selenium: Increases natural killer cells and cancer fighting cells. There is some promising evidence of its cancer prevention abilities.

- Omega-3 fatty acids: Is a very beneficial fat. It is anti- inflammatory, associated with good heart health, boosts immune system especially the phagocytes, and has anti-cancer effects.

- Mushrooms: Known for centuries to have immune boosting qualities in the Orient. Maitake, Reishi, and Shiitake strengthen the immune system and fight diseases like cancer.

FOODS THAT PROMOTEIN FLAMMATION

"The more severe the pain or illness, the more severe will be the necessary changes. These may involve breaking bad habits, or acquiring some new and better ones." -Peter McWilliams

You are not helpless in your fight against inflammation! Your diet plays a major role in activating or suppressing a protein called cytokines that causes inflammation. I can't stress this enough. For that and other reasons that will be discussed shortly, I would like you to start thinking in terms of: "Is what I'm swallowing making me healthier or sicker?" There is little if any neutral ground. It is as if everything that you swallow is sending a signal to your immune system to either cause more inflammation or less.

The following are groups of foods that you should avoid because they send a signal to your body to produce more inflammatory cytokines. They are also toxic to your body in multiple ways, polluting the internal terrain of the body and promoting inflammation.

Most Meat, Except Oily Fish

We often hear the phrase "all things in moderation". Meat, especially red meat, is an exception to this rule.

Even what most would consider a "moderate" amount of red meat can produce an intolerable number of cytokines and bring on autoimmune symptoms.

For some, the "low-carb craze" has meant an increase in meat consumption. If eating the low-carb way means that you are eating a lot of meat, you are making your autoimmune condition worse. Protein from meat raises the levels of the toxins uric acid and urea in the blood. The body pumps excessive amounts of water into the kidneys to help flush out these toxins. The result of a high animal-based protein diet is very quick water "weight loss". The downside of this "weight loss" is that it causes the body to lose essential minerals. Mineral deficiencies cause autoimmunity. A better protein choice comes from vegetable-based proteins. These proteins improve mineral retention in the body.

One doctor has reported that within two weeks of his lupus patients not eating meat, most showed significant improvement in their skin lesions.

The Swank Diet calls for giving up red meat for one year. Then, after the first year, allowing yourself four ounces of red meat per week. This diet has made a significant improvement in the lives of people with Multiple Sclerosis (MS). Dr. Swank studied more than 150 of his patients with MS for a thirty-four year period of time. Those who followed the diet died at the rate of 5%, while patients not following his diet had a death rate of about 85% during the same time period.

However, reducing meat intake isn't just about living longer, it is about living well! This recommendation is for everyone, not just those whose collection of autoimmune symptoms are called lupus or MS. No matter where in your body cytokines gather or what they are attacking, eating red meat will increase their numbers. The way that meat is prepared also makes a difference. Charbroiled and grilled meats of any kind are much worse for you and should be completely avoided.

Fish is the exception to the meat rule. Fish does not raise cytokine levels. It actually reduces them. The problem is that much of our fish is contaminated with toxic mercury. Unless you are sure that your fish source is mercury free, you should limit your fish intake to one serving per week and use fish oil supplements instead. Some people will even be sensitive to one contaminated serving of fish. Check your local health food stores for fish farmed in "mercury-free" tested water. Additionally, salmon is a fish that is readily available and least likely to be mercury contaminated.

Egg Yolks

Egg yolks and dairy products are high in arachidonic acid. This is the same substance that makes meats so inflammatory. If you are going to eat eggs, you should only eat the whites. On a food label, eggs can be listed as albumin, globulin, ovamucin, or vitellin.

Dairy Products

"...countries with the highest dairy consumption, such as the United States and Sweden, because of their high animal protein diets, have the highest rates of osteoporosis, a disease involving the weakening and potential breaking of bones."

Research published in the Lancet Medical Journal described a small group of patients with Chronic Fatigue Syndrome (CFS) in Norway. For four years, they experienced substantial improvement by excluding milk and wheat from their diets. Reintroducing these foods into their diets caused a significant rise in the patients' cytokine levels along with an increase in pain.

Besides increasing cytokines, milk further aggravates asthma because of its casein content. When the protein of another animal is introduced into the human body, the immune system responds with an allergic reaction. Casein is a milk protein. Eating casein causes your body to produce histamines, which result in excess mucus production.

Those with CFS and asthma are not alone in their sensitivity to milk. According to the New England Journal of Medicine, July 30, 1992, studies suggest that a certain milk protein is responsible for the onset of diabetes because patients produce antibodies to cow milk proteins.

Milk's vices are many. As strange as it may sound, the digestion of milk proteins can create an addictive substance that acts like endorphins, our own personal narcotics. The same can be true of gluten and wheat. These endorphins have the ability to disrupt brain chemistry and cause addiction.

I am sorry, but this has to be said: Last year, the average liter of milk in America contained 323 million pus cells. Sick and infected cowshave cell counts above 200 million. A count of 323 million is not even healthy by dairy industry standards. Drinking pus is a bad idea for anyone. Itis a terrible idea for someone with a tendency towards immune dysfunction.

Gluten

Gluten is a component of grains such as wheat, oats, barley, and rye. Besides being inflammatory, doctors have reported a higher than average number of people with autoimmune disorders are allergic to gluten. They suggest complete avoidance for at least one month to see if benefits will occur.

Studies have also shown that wheat and corn can irritate patients with Rheumatoid Arthritis and raise cytokine production in the colon and rectum of those with celiac disease.

Corn, Corn Oil, Corn Syrup (Fructose)

Corn, besides promoting cytokines, has been called the leading cause of chronic food addiction in this century. To give you an idea of how powerful the addiction can be, all cigarettes made in the U.S. since World War I have contained added sugars, usually from corn. Do you think the cigarette companies chose corn syrup for the great taste it adds to their products?

Corn syrup (fructose) is cheap and twice as sweet as cane sugar. In 1994, the average person ate 83 pounds of fructose. Corn syrup causes an increase in blood lactic acid, especially in people with diabetes. Fructose from corn syrup inhibits copper metabolism and decreases mineral availability, two factors in autoimmunity. Fructose also breaks down into a substance that weakens your body's natural anti- inflammatory molecules. The body does not metabolize fructose the same as other sugars. Fructose converts to fat more than any other sugar. Corn fructose certainly isn't the diabetic-friendly and harmless sugar substitute that it is advertised to be.

Studies have shown that corn can irritate patients with Rheumatoid Arthritis (RA) and the National Fibromyalgia Association (NFA) suggests corn should be avoided because it can aggravate Fibromyalgia.

Remember that if corn products can increase cytokine levels in those with RA and Fibromyalgia, it can increase cytokine levels for anyone.

Sugar

We Americans are eating an average of 153 pounds of sugar a year.

Refined white sugar makes

it more difficult for your body to absorb vitamins and minerals, a major contributor to the cause of autoimmunity. Sugar also suppresses immune function, leaving us open to infection. Just eight tablespoons of sugar, which is the equivalent to the sugar in less than one 12-ounce can of soda, can reduce the ability of your immune system to kill germs by up to 40%.

Like salt, sugar is dehydrating to the body. Dehydration increases histamine, which can

worsen asthma and any other autoimmune disease because histamine increases cytokine production. As recommend by the National Fibromyalgia Association (NFA), sugars should be avoided because they can worsen the condition. Sugar feeds Lyme-causing bacteria and Candida yeast, the significance of which will be discussed later. Eating sugar also causes an insulin surge, which contributes to chronic inflammation.

Honey is sugar. It may be "all natural", but it is still sugar. It is higher in calories than table sugar and can be contaminated by pesticides. Consuming "all natural" delicious tasting pesticides is not what you want to be doing.

A good non-toxic substitute for sugar is the nutritional supplement stevia. Stevia has been used by millions of people without reported side effects. In Japan, stevia sweetened products represent 41% of the market share of sweet substances consumed.

Stevia is an herb originally from Paraguay. South Americans use it as a sweetener and also for medicinal purposes. This herb is anywhere from 30 to 100 times sweeter than sugar. Stevia does not affect the blood sugar levels of most diabetics. Stevia also does not feed fungus in the intestines like sugars do.

Stevia has a strong, sweet flavor that can overwhelm a recipe, so it should be used sparingly. Because you only use such a small amount at a time, recipes must be adjusted for the lack of bulk. Stevia can often be purchased with helpful inulin added to it for bulk. Also, cakes and cookies sweetened with stevia do not brown as much as their sugar- sweetened counterparts.

Flour/Processed Foods

For you simple carbohydrate-lovers (addicts), the next

sentence is going to be one of the most painful ones in the book. If you want to get ridof cytokine inflammation, you must give up processed foods and junk foods. They tend to be full of everything you shouldn't eat. This list includes most breakfast cereals, muffins, breads, crackers, cookies, and doughnuts.

White flour contains alloxan, which is the chemical used to make flour look clean and white. Alloxan destroys the insulin-producing beta cells of the pancreas. It does so by initiating free radical damage to the DNA in the pancreas. Researchers believe that some people have weak defenses to free radicals in these beta cells. Alloxan is so potent that researchers who study diabetes use it to give diabetes to lab animals. While not everyone who eats white breads and processed foods will get diabetes, the connection is clear: Alloxan causes diabetes in those genetically susceptible to the disease.

The Nightshade Family

Vegetables in the nightshade family include white potatoes, tomatoes, all peppers, cherries, tobacco, and eggplants. Research indicates that these vegetables produce pain and inflammation in arthritis patients and aggravate Fibromyalgia according to the National Fibromyalgia Association (NFA). However, not everyone will be sensitive to nightshade foods. The only way to know for sure is to avoid them for a period of weeks then reintroduce them into your diet.

Everyone should avoid tobacco, which is a toxic member of the nightshade family, permanently.

Coffee

Despite being inflammatory, coffee has had its medicinal purposes. My own ancestors used it to treat asthma. I have friends outside the U.S., who are still dependent upon coffee to treat asthma. Certain caffeine-type chemicals in coffee have been proven effective at stimulating bronchial dilation in people diagnosed with specific types of asthma. Some modern day asthma medications are even made from chemicals in the caffeine family.

For those using coffee as a natural asthma medication, you should keep in mind that caffeine is a toxic chemical. Its purpose in plant life is to act as an insecticide. In people, caffeine suppresses the enzymes needed for memory making. It also raises both blood sugar and insulin levels, causing cytokine production and aggravating diabetes.

Simply drinking decaffeinated coffee isn't the answer either. Women who drink more than one cup a day of decaffeinated coffee are considered at a much higher risk of developing rheumatoid arthritis. The theory is that chemically decaffeinated products are causing the increased risk of autoimmunity. If you are going to drink decaffeinated coffee anyway, be sure that it uses a non-chemical based decaffeinating method and that the coffee was organically grown. Those who do not drink organic coffee, are exposed to too many man-made pesticides.

Alcohol

The wine industry has America convinced that a glass or two a day is good for your heart. However, John Folts, Ph.D of the University of Wisconsin, has done studies, which show that to receive those heart- healthy benefits, you would have to consume enough wine to be declared legally drunk. Grape juice is a healthier alternative. Dr. Folt's study also found that only ten to twelve ounces of purple grape juice was associated with lower blood clotting, thus a lower risk of heart disease than promised by red wine.

Besides being pro-inflammatory and addictive, alcohol breaks down to a toxin in the body called aldehyde. Toxins are dangerous chemicals that the liver does not recognize as useful. Toxins attack and destroy cells and attract germs. Aldehyde accumulates in the brain, spinal cord, joints, muscles and tissues, where it causes muscle weakness, irritation, and pain.

BENEFITS OF ANTI-INFLAMMATORY SUPPLEMENTS

Anti Inflammatory Supplements may offer some relief for those who suffer from the painful effects of inflammation. Inflammation can result in heat, pain, redness and swelling and can target specific areas of the body including the bladder, gums, prostate, sinuses and skin. However, it can also affect the entire body. You can use natural Anti Inflammatory Supplements to help keep the condition under control without suffering the effects of stomach ulcers that can come with prescription medication or NSAIDS. You may already be familiar with many of these types of supplements, and you may even be taking some already.

For instance, more people are becoming aware of fish oil supplements. There are many benefits to fish oil, but its primary appeal is that it is rich in omega-3 fatty acids. These fatty acids are beneficial to those suffering from inflammation because they reduce the body'sproduction of inflammatory biochemicals. It also decreases the amount of interleukins, which signifies chronic inflammation. Those suffering from arthritis may also reduce their dosage of anti-inflammatory drugs if fish oil works for them. The downside to fish oil is that when you first begin to use it, you may tend to belch up a fish taste for a short time after taking them. For this reason, many take the supplements little by little throughout the day to decrease that particular side effect.

Zinc can also be used as Anti Inflammatory Supplements to fight inflammation in addition to its immune system boosting properties. Zinc can reduce an inflammation increasing cytokine called TNF-alpha. Zinc is found prevalently in poultry, red meat and sea foods. However, you can also get them from beans, cereals, dairy products, nuts and whole grains. When you do not absorb enough zinc from food, you may have to take supplements. The most common side effect from supplements is zinc overdose. You should not take more than 40 milligrams of zinc per day.

Antioxidants are good for more than skin care. Antioxidants can fight inflammation by helping to reduce the oxidative damage that comes when immune cells fight infection. You may already be familiar with

many antioxidants such as selenium, vitamin C and vitamin E. They neutralize the free radicals that cause oxidative damage. However, you should avoid consuming too many antioxidants. This can result in mild and severe effects including reduced muscle function, weakened immune system, toxic reactions and risk of heart failure.

HEART ATTACK AND HEART DISEASE TRIGGERED BY INFLAMMATION

Doctors and researchers have recently made great new strides in our quest to understand, protect against and eventually eliminate heart disease.

Numerous studies reported in prestigious medical journals now identify INFLAMMATION, not cholesterol, as the major culprit in causing heart disease, and as it turns out, inflammation can be accurately measured by a simple test that costs under $50.

Research studies that number in the thousands and continue to this day show that INFLAMMATION plays a much bigger role in triggering heart attacks and heart disease than cholesterol.

These studies show that people with normal cholesterol AND high levels of a substance called C-reactive protein, which measuresinflammation, are at greater risk of heart attack than people with high cholesterol and normal levels of CRP.

What is C-reactive protein? C-reactive protein, (CRP) is one of a number of molecules produced by the immune system for the specific purpose of containing or repairing artery damage that occurs for a variety of different reasons.

Discovering the connection between inflammation and heart disease is a MAJOR ADVANCE in understanding the disease. And the ease with which C-reactive protein can be measured gives doctors a powerful new tool to identify high-risk individuals who, other than elevated CRP, have no other heart disease risk factors.

Cholesterol has always had much more press than it deserves.

While it's true that about half of the people with heart disease have high cholesterol, it is also true about half the people with heart diseasehave

NORMAL cholesterol, which means cholesterol may NOT be a significant causal factor.

The new research on inflammation and the role of C-reactive protein is so compelling that many doctors now believe the evidence is overwhelming and that inflammation is, with total certainty, thecentral factor in cardiovascular disease.

The bottom line is this; the next time you have a check up be sure and have your C-reactive protein tested because this test, exclusive of all others, provides objective information about your risk of heart disease that is far more important than any other factor capable of being tested at this time, including cholesterol.

Causes Of Inflammation And Increased C-Reactive Protein

Here is what we know. When cells that line the inside of the arteries are injured or become dysfunctional they send out a signal, kind of like an SOS, a cry for help. The cellular distress signals are heard by the immune system and the immune system answers the distress call by sending in specialized cells and molecules, including C-reactive protein, to contain the injury, repair the damage and fight off the offender.

If you take a beautiful landscape, like the inside of a healthy artery, and turn it into a war zone where damage and injury is occurring and special troops are being poured in by the thousands to attack the enemy and contain the damage, it does not take long before the landscape is not so pretty anymore.

We know inflammation causes big problems, but what causes

inflammation?

What damages the inside of the artery in the first place?

What causes the cells to cry for help and get the immune system, to send in the shock troops in the form of C-reactive protein and other substances?

We don't know everything that causes damage inside the artery walls, but here are a few things we do know.

Basically ANYTHING that causes injury or inflammation signals the release of powerful immune system substances for the purpose of containing and repairing the damage and attacking the problem. So what causes inflammation?

Tobacco is a brutal toxin. Smoking litters the blood with powerful chemicals that damage artery walls and stimulate an immune system response, which, if maintained over time, causes the build up of inflammatory chemicals and greatly increases the risk of heart attack and heart disease.

Both high blood pressure and diabetes put constant stress on the inside of the artery walls. Elevated levels of C-reactive protein are common in people with either of these problems.

Although researchers are not certain as to why, we know that certain medicines cause an elevation of C-reactive protein, which is another good reason to get healthy, stay healthy and not depend on medicines of any sort.

Infections signal the immune system to release C-reactive protein. Many people suffer with low-grade infections that constantly sap their energy. Often, these people have no idea they are suffering with infections; they just think theyre tired.

Inflammation causes inflammation. You read it right, theres no misprint. The inflammatory chemicals produced by the immune system and sent into the blood to contain damage, repair damage and fight invaders actually become part of the problem IF the cellular call for help never stops.

Think about it, if storm troopers constantly trample through your garden, how will it ever grow back and be nice again? The answer is, it won't!

These are a few of the OBVIOUS causes of inflammation. Now lets examine sources of inflammation that are not so obvious and potentially even more dangerous because they are likely to go unrecognized.

Does being overweight CAUSE inflammation?

Until recently researchers believed that fat cells were passive, but new research has proven differently. It turns out that fat cells are not at all passive.

Fat cells constantly produce a substance called interleukin-6.

Interleukin-6 is a highly specialized, extremely powerful, pro- inflammatory bio-chemical that can cause great damage if it shows up in the body at the wrong place and for the wrong reasons. AND FAT CELLS MAKE IT

ALL THE TIME.

Interleukin-6 is like a pack of vicious attack dogs your immune system can set lose against viruses, tumors, or anything that may seriously threaten your health. But if there are no bad guys to attack, the last thing a peaceful neighborhood needs is a band of killer dogs roaming the streets ready to pounce on anything that moves.

When interleukin-6 enters the blood it does exactly what it is meant to do. It attacks.

Interleukin-6 causes an immediate inflammatory response, damaging cells and creating problems.

The injured cells send out a distress signal and the liver responds by making C-reactive protein and sending it streaming into the blood to solve a problem that never ends as long as interleukin-6 is present.

Because of the never ending supply of interleukin-6 that fat cells so graciously provide, overweight individuals live in a state of constant low- grade inflammation, which keeps C-reactive protein high and dramatically raises the risk of heart disease.

Now you understand exactly why losing weight slows the inflammation process, lowers C-reactive protein in the body and reduces the risk of heart disease. And you understand even better why losing weight and

firming up is one of the healthiest things you can

possibly do for yourself. See you at the gym!

Do Sugar And Carbohydrates CAUSE Artery Damage & Inflammation?

Make no mistake about it. Over consumption of foods high in sugar and carbohydrates is one of the primary initiating causes of hypertension, heart disease, diabetes, kidney failure, gall bladder disease and about half of all cancers.

Besides causing metabolic imbalances that can destroy your health in a variety of different and creative ways, sugar and carbohydrates turn into glucose and glucose auto-oxidizes in your blood, spinning off free radicals that damage the artery, cause inflammation and send your cells screaming for help.

The ramifications of this are staggering, especially in light of the new research that shows INFLAMMATION to be the primary underlying cause of heart disease.

The health destructive effects of oxidation and free radicals are well documented in medical literature. In fact, research on free radicals is one of the main reasons supplements known as ANTI OXIDANTS are so popular.

Nutrients like vitamin c, selenium and zinc are important because they are powerful anti-oxidants that help protect against oxidative stress and free radical damage.

Here are the facts. Decide for yourself.

FACT: Sugar and carbohydrates are converted into glucose and glucose quickly enters your blood and raises your blood sugar.

FACT: Glucose auto oxidizes in the blood causing significant free radical production.

FACT: Free radicals rip and slice the arteries, causing damage, producing inflammation and causing the cells to cry for help.C-reactive

protein is made in the liver and sent charging into the blood to answer the call.

The bottom line . . .

Eating a diet high in sugar or carbohydrates keeps blood glucose levels high resulting in oxidative stress, free radical production, arterial damage, a cellular cry for help and an accommodating liver that makes C-reactive protein to answer the call.

If you believe the latest research about inflammation and heart disease, and most cardiologist in America do, then you have to agree that eating a diet high in sugar and carbohydrates is a PERFECT PRESCRIPTION for developing heart disease.

REAL STRESS RELIEF SOLUTION

The Shocking Truth that Stress and Inflammation- not your Genes- Control your Destiny!

Proven tips and strategies to STOP IT!

Diet and exercise control something called inflammation - which is born from stress. Now if there is no stress in your life, then you don't have to read the rest of this article.

Where you aware that inflammation is the possible cause of 80 - 90% of diseases in the body? Another way of saying this is to say that the reaction the body has to un-channeled, unfocused chronic stress is synonymous with inflammation. This low-grade inflammation that very people think about, know about, is the demise of our health!

Stress/inflammation can lead into such common disease as Alzheimer's, allergies, Arthritis (yes, all of the over 100 types), heart disease, MS, cancer, IBS, ulcers, skin disorders, migraines - and the list goes on.

All of this research point to one simple fact: the medical/research community is baffled by the complete process of inflammation.

This ebook is not to give you a crash chemistry lesson,

but to assure you that one of the most profound answers to 21st century health care is much simpler than you think. Well, in that simplicity - it reveals ultra complexity!

In my research and in my own experience of surviving cancer, autoimmune disorders, arthritis, and multiple surgeries and infections from those surgeries, I am here to tell you that nothing......Nothing....will ever help you to heal and recuperate your health more than training the mind/body with the easiest being exercise or movement based therapies.

Genes aren't your Destiny!

If fact if you have a disease - you can guarantee that inflammation from stress plays a huge part in its development and/or exacerbation. And no, you can't just blame your genes anymore. Genetics plays less than 20% of your disease. Genes are not your destiny...!!!

Emotions, Diet, exercise (or the lack thereof), and stress control your destiny!

In other words, your mind...or your reactions to your internal /external environment - processed by the mind are your destiny.

Movement is key to a healthy mind and body. Bodhidharma, way back in the 5th and 6th century found this out when the monks he was trying to teach to become enlightened by meditation, could not hold a single point thought because their body was so deconditioned. Your body is designed to move, work and then rest and relax or meditate - a Yin / Yang balance.

The Life History of Inflammation

A brief summary of how inflammation starts and continues in thebody:

- Stress causes an increased output of cortisol from the adrenal glands which fuels inflammation.

- Lack of sleep places a stress on the body with an inability to recuperate from previous days stressors.

- Too much fat, sugar, preservatives, processed and fast foods, sodas and energy drinks as well as over-proportioned amounts of fatty meat.

- An imbalance of organisms in your gut causes your immune system to overreact. H pylori is a bacteria in the stomach that contributes to inflammation and the development of ulcers. H pylori is present in 50% of adults over 60 years old and in 20%of adults under the age of 40!

- Leaky gut - an increase in the permeability of the intestinal lining can result in toxins leaking from the bowel resulting in inflammation

- Chronic low-grade food allergies or food sensitivities that may cause few symptoms.

- Toxins from food, water, your environment and personal care products. Most folks never think about the products they rub on their skin, but much of that can be absorbed into the blood.

- Food sensitivity or intolerance and food allergies cause low grade

- inflammation

- Obesity - the fatty tissues of the body secrete hormones that regulate the immune system and inflammation, but in the case of an overweight individual this can become out of control.

- Dehydration makes inflammation worse So what can we do?

- Well start by including the following foods.

10 excellent inflammation-fighting foods

- Long Grain rice (Basmati, Jasmine etc) are really good for helping quiet inflammation and is a great alternative to the enormous amount of wheat product we consume

- Wild caught salmon, not farm-raised salmon, is

another way to get beneficial omega-3 fatty acids. You can also try other fatty fish like mackerel and sardines.

- Tart cherries can reduce inflammation ten times better than aspirin! Tart cherries or cherry juice help reduce your risk for heart

- disease. Tart Cherry juice is also good to drink for bladder infections and UTI's.

- Walnuts are often mentioned, but I have found a lot of folks allergic to this nut. A better choice is chestnuts roasted.

- Onions and Garlic. Onions have lots of quercetin, a potent antioxidant that can help your body fight inflammation. Becareful with onions if you have an irritable gut. Garlic has long been a folk remedy for colds and illness, and its anti-inflammatory properties are spectacular. Again be careful not to eat too much at once until you know your tolerance. Also, fresh garlic needs to be mashedin order for it to become biologically active with its anti-inflammatory properties.

- Fermented Foods and Liquids like organic Keefer, Yogurt and raw milk are good for the gut. If the gut is happy, your body is happy!

- Spices: Ginger & Tumeric

Turmeric is a spice used extensively in other cultures, and for good reason. It contains curcumin, a substance that actively reduces inflammation.

Ginger works in a way similar to tumeric to lower inflammation and in some studies has been shown to reduce pain associated with arthritis.

Next...GO FOR A WALK!!!

Yes..this is the oldest form of exercise and is probably the best and always will be. Take your dog for a walk and then pet the dog - all has been proven to lower blood pressure and the inflammation response!

CHRONIC INFLAMMATION CAN CAUSE SERIOUS HARM TO YOUR BODY

Inflammation touches many aspects of our life. It plays an important role in our body, and it's not something we can do without. But even as it protects us and plays a critical role when we are injured, it can cause problems if it gets out of control. When this happens we refer to it as chronic inflammation.

It may seem a little strange that something so important to our well- being and good health can also ruin our health, and even cause death, but it is true. Chronic inflammation is something you definitely want to avoid.

Heart disease and cancer have both been linked to problems with inflammation. In relation to heart disease, it can cause coronary blockage, and a heart attack. We've been told for years to keep our cholesterol low to avoid the buildup of plaque in our arteries, but scientist now believe that inflammation may play as important a roleas cholesterol and plaque.

Inflammation is also a villain in relation to cancer, particularly in the initiation of cancer. Things are not as clear here, and certainly not all cancers are caused by inflammation. Nevertheless some of the cells and chemicals involved in inflammation have been shown to create mutations in DNA that can eventually lead to cancer; furthermore, it can also cause pre-cancer cells to become active cancer cells. A few of the cancers known to be associated with inflammation are colon, lung, stomach, esophagus, and breast cancer.

Many other diseases are also associated with inflammation. Rheumatoid arthritis, osteoporosis, MS, lupus, emphysema, and gingivitis are all inflammation diseases. Indeed, any disease with a name with "it is" at the end of it is an inflammatory disease. A few examples are: bursitis, tendonitis, arthritis, hepatitis, colitis, tonsillitis, and dermatitis.

How Inflammation Begins and Proceeds

Inflammation is the response of the body to harmful stimuli. Several things that can initiate it are:

- Infection by pathogens (bacteria, viruses and so on)

- Physical injury

- Foreign bodies that enter body such as splinters, dirt or other

- debris

- Chemical irritants

- Burns and frostbite

- Stress

- Toxins from air or water

Everyone has experienced inflammation in one form or another. It's major symptoms are redness, swelling, heat and pain. In most cases, however, what we experience is acute inflammation. It is a short term process lasting only a few days to a few weeks, and in most cases it ceases when the stimuli is removed. So for most people it is not serious. Chronic inflammation, on the other hand, is inflammation that does not clear up properly. It persists for months, and sometimes, years. And it can do considerable harm to your body. This articles is mainly concerned with chronic inflammation.

We'll begin, however, with an overview of acute inflammation. It goes through two main phases: a vascular phase and a cellular phase. And it consists of a series of biochemical events that involve the local vascular system, the immune system and cells within the injured tissue. A brief (and simplified) outline of how it takes place is as follows:

- The process begins when a harmful stimuli of some sort is detected.

- The initial response (vascular phase) comes from immune system cells present in the affected tissue. One of the major ones that detects it first and reacts is called macrophages. They have receptors that recognize pathogens and other foreign objects (not belonging to the body).

- These macrophages (and other particles) release inflammation mediators that call in other particles. They also release mediator molecules, including histamine, that dilate the blood vessels in the vicinity. This increases the blood flow to the affected area; it also increases the permeability (leakage) of these vessels.

- The increased blood flow allows more infection-fighting immune cells to reach the area. It also increases the amount of glucose (sugar) and oxygen to the area to help nourish the cells. At the same time the increased permeability of the vessels helps bring in plasma protein and fluids that contain antibodies and so on to the area.

- As a result of the above the affected area swells and turns red. There is also some heating and there may be pain.

- The cellular phase begins as the increased size of the blood vessels helps the migration of white blood cells, mainly neutrophils and macrophages, into the area. They are particularly important when pathogens are present, in that they eat them, but they also perform other important roles such as assisting in repair of the wound.

- One of the main things the above buildup does is "wall off" the area from further attack, particularly from bacteria and viruses.

- When the pathogen (or whatever) is overcome a cleanup of dead cells and other debris begins. The initiation of a process where new, healthy cells replace the old ones begins, and soon the macrophages and other immune cells leave the area. And in the acute case everything soon gets back to normal.

Chronic Inflammation

Unfortunately everything doesn't always go as smoothly as described in the above process. Several things can go wrong, and when they do, serious problems can occur. (Thankfully, this doesn't happen too often.)

The major problem is usually associated with the termination of the inflammation. In particular, the attack on the foreign objects doesn't stop as it should. Macrophages and other particles may be left behind and they can do considerable damage to healthy tissue. One reason this might happen is that these particles check a "password" on the surface of cells and if it is a normal body cell they ignore it, but if it is foreign they attack it. Sometimes, however,the password system breaks down and the immune cells mistake body cells for intruders and destroy them. This leads to what is called autoimmune disease (such as lupus and MS).

In the same way, allergies of various types can occur when the immune system overacts. Pollens are usually considered harmless by the immune system, but in some cases it can suddenly decide they are dangerous and attack them. The result may be asthma.

Or the immune system may see damage due to LDL cholesterol in the arteries as a problem and try to repair it. As a result the immune cells become bloated and stick to the sides of the arteries creating plaque.

Most changes of this type occur when a person has a weakened immune system so it it's easy to see why a strong immune system is important.

Who is Most at Risk

First of all it's important to point out that everyone needs to be concerned about inflammation getting out of control, and everyone should do what they can to strengthen their immune system. Nevertheless, there are things that make some people more prone to chronic inflammation and other inflammation problems. They are:

- Anyone who is overweight (in particular, obese). The immune system frequently mistakes fat deposits for intruders and attacks them. In addition, fat cells can leak or break open; if this happens macrophages come in to clear up the debris, and they may release chemicals that cause problems.

- Anyone with diabetes. Studies show that diabetes II may be related to inflammation, and that people with high levels of inflammation usually develop diabetes within a few years.

- Anyone with symptoms of heart disease or heart disease in the family. There are several relationships between heart disease and chronic inflammation. Also, it's well-known that the plaque in arteries, which results from inflammation, causes heart attacks.

- Anyone who feels tired and fatigued all the time. This is particularly important if no reason can be found for the problem. Fatigue is associated with inflammation.

- Anyone who works in a toxic environment. It's well known that toxins cause excess inflammation.

- Any one suffering extensively from depression or anxiety. It's well- known that stress causes inflammation.

- Older People. Our body changes as we age and we tend to produce more pro-inflammation chemicals and fewer anti-inflammation chemicals.

What You can do to Avoid Chronic Inflammation

The above list should give you a good idea what to do to avoid chronic inflammation, nevertheless I'll list some of the major things and briefly discuss them. I should mention, however, that genes play a role in whether or not you'll get chronic inflammation, and there's little we can do about them.

A list of the major things is as follows:

- Eat a highly nutritious diet. It should include at least five servings of vegetables and fruit each day. Cruciferous vegetables are particularly important; they include broccoli, cauliflower, and cabbage. Other excellent vegetables are carrots, tomatoes, spinach and beans. Some of the best fruits are citrus fruits; berries such as blueberries and strawberries are also important. Other things that are particularly good are grains such as oats and whole wheat, nuts and seeds. Fish is also important as a source of

- omega-3, and you should eat it 2 to 3 times a week. At the same time you should avoid simple carbohydrates, fast foods, soda, saturated fats and trans fat products.

- Don't overeat. Also, if you are over-weight, lose weight.

- Get sufficient sleep. For most adults 7 to 8 hours is sufficient.

- Exercise regularly. Exercise is, in fact, a good way to lower inflammation. Both aerobic and weights are important.

- Control your cholesterol, blood pressure and triglycerides.

- Avoid stress.

- Avoid toxins.

HIDDEN BENEFITS OF ANTI-INFLAMMATORY FISH OIL

Most people don't know this but inflammation in our bodies can be a silent killer. It can cause heart disease and other serious illness over the long run. We all have it to some extent but it's hard to tell so we may not even know it.

Oftentimes, however, even if it's not causing serious disease, it shows up in the form of other troubling problems that can make life miserable. But, anti inflammatory fish oil can help reduce inflammation-related health problems.

While the dangerous health effects of inflammation are only beginning to be widely understood, the value of taking high-quality pure fish oil is well-researched and proven. In fact, for heart disease, you could experience more advantages from taking an anti inflammatory fish oil than you do aspirin if you take the right product.

So, what kinds inflammation can pure fish oil combat? Well, we've already mentioned inflammation that causes heart disease that many people take aspirin to combat. But, while aspirin can hurt your stomach, for those in good digestive health, the right fish oil shouldn't bother your stomach at all.

But, even if you have an inflammatory bowel disorder like ulcerative colitis or Crohn's disease, studies show high-quality fish oil supplements can help you. Fish oil has been shown to reduce painful inflammation associated with Crohn's disease. In fact, 69% of those who took it in studies stay symptom free compared to 28% of those who took a placebo.

Similarly, instead of taking drugs like aspirin for arthritis, you might be able to take omega-3 supplements. Research proves that these supplements, particularly when they're the highest quality, are very helpful in reducing arthritic symptoms. That could increase your ability to move around substantially if you have RA (rheumatoid arthritis) by making it less painful.

These products also help gout by reducing the compounds in your bloodstream that lead to gout.

And, if you have skin problems like psoriasis and acne, omega-3 fatty acids also help improve the quality and health of skin. Using pure fish oil reduces the inflammation associated with these conditions and fights the effects of skin inflammation caused by aging, too.

But, most people's biggest concern around aging still remains heart disease because it's the number one killer in the United States. Every 25 seconds, an American will have a coronary event and many won't survive. Moreover, a lot of times, people have no idea that this disease, aggravated by inflammation, is plaguing them. High-quality, anti inflammatory fish oil has been shown to help significantly reduce heart disease.

Now, these pills aren't a cure for heart disease and, alone, won't prevent it. But coupled with a healthy diet and weight as well as moderate exercise, omega-3 fatty acids can go a long way in decreasing your chances of a deadly heart attacks and increasing overall heart health.

So, now you're convinced. Inflammation is a big health problem that can be dangerous and omega-3 fatty acids can significantly reduce the health dangers connected with it. Well, what do you need to do next?

You must do own your research. But, keep some things in mind when you do.

For the most benefit, make sure the product you purchase can actually give you the most anti inflammatory fish oil per pill available for your money.

Also, make sure they're not only made from the purest fish oils from the best sources but are mostly free of contaminants and fillers. Your supplements should be consistently fresh, and should be tested and guaranteed to be exactly that.

By making certain of these things, you're sure to find your fish oil supplements won't do more harm than good. And, buying the best quality anti inflammatory fish oil is

sure to give you your desired results and enhance your
health.

THE MOST COMMON CAUSES OF INFLAMMATION AND THE RELATIONSHIP TO GUT HEALTH

We hear a lot about inflammation these days.

In a clinical setting, we've been talking about inflammation to our practice members for years. Along with toxicity, stress, and deficiency, inflammation is at the very heart of the causes of chronic illness and dysfunction.

However, I've noticed an interesting shift recently. We've got people seeking care for various reasons, who will tell us things like, "At times, I feel completely inflamed... like that's what's causing my problems. But my (conventional) doctor thinks I'm nuts!"

(Or, even worse, they're put on anti-inflammatory medication or steroids as a result of expressing their concerns to their doc.)

It's an intriguing time as a growing number of independent health seekers are searching for the root causes to their afflictions.

When we talk about inflammation, by the way, we're talking about systemic inflammation - cellular inflammation. It's not the same as twisting your ankle and then witnessing the localized swelling that results.

182

The inflammation we're talking about here is far more insidious. It's like a chronic irritant to our bodies and minds... like a fire quietly raging within.

It's of particular importance to address inflammation of the gut. The gut is intricately tied to the brain and brain function, as cutting-edge scientific research continues to demonstrate. A "bad gut equals a bad brain". Consider the potential for more accurately and successfully treating (or preventing) conditions like depression, anxiety, spectrum disorders, Alzheimer's, and so on. The gut must not be overlooked.

So, what causes inflammation? Lots.

Here are some of the most common factors associated with inflammation:

1. Diet - Eating "inflammatory" foods, especially grains like wheat, barley, and rye that contain gluten and introduce inflammatory proteins called prolamins. These chronically irritate the gut and contribute to gut permeability or "leaky gut". Once the gut is excessively permeable, large molecules that were never intended to pass through the intestinal barrier are allowed to do so. This triggers an over-active immune response as the immune system goes on the attack, so to speak. One of the results of this heightened immune reaction is inflammation.

2. Sugar - Whether it's the white powdery, crystal stuff right off the spoon or right out of a packet, or it's foods and drinks that break down to sugar rapidly in our bloodstream (like juice, pop, sweets and starchy carbs like bread, pasta, cereal, crackers, pizza, baked goods & pastries) sugar spikes create a negative response across the board. Blood sugar dysregulation from chronic sugar spikes and insulin resistance are direct contributors to inflammation. Artificial sweeteners are clearly not a solution! These are highly toxic and contribute to inflammation as well.

3. "Bad" Fats - Another dietary culprit. These are the trans fats, hydrogenated & partially hydrogenated fats, commercial vegetable oils, the fat from contaminated animal sources, excess omega-6 fats & oils, and so on. These contribute to an inflammatory condition. Stick with pure coconut oil, real grass-fed butter, organic extra virgin olive oil, healthy fats from grass-fed & free-range animal sources, wild fish, healthy fat foods like avocado, a balance of omega-3 to omega-6 fats, and so on. The "bad" fats are typically what we get with junk food, fast food, restaurant food, fried foods, and so forth. Even when we start with "healthy" food, when we cook

it with bad fats, the results are toxic and inflammatory.

4. Leaky Gut & Autoimmune Conditions - I know I just mentioned it, but it needs its own distinct place on this list. It's a vicious cycle: leaky gut leads to inflammation... which leads to leaky gut... which leads to more

5. inflammation. You get the point. This is an immune response, actually. The immune system is simply doing its job of attacking things that aren't supposed to be there, like too-large molecules passing through the intestinal barrier. When this cycle continues, the stage is perfectly set for an autoimmune condition as the immune response continues on its attack "against" the body. The intelligent approach to correcting this is NOT to suppress the overall immune response, but to (1) remove the triggers, thereby 'calming' the immune response, and (2) heal the gut.

6. Stress - Whether it's mental, emotional, or physical, chronic stress plays a direct role in cellular inflammation. Our bodies are perfectly suited to short bouts with stress - it's called the "fight or flight response". But, when we're chronically exposed to stress, systems break down. This can be from ongoing financial issues,

185

relationship challenges, career dissatisfaction, chronic sleep deprivation, injury, over-working, over-training (e.g. for a marathon), drugs, toxic foods... there's no shortage of stressors! Stress creates a unique cascade of neuro-hormonal events in the brain and body that simply cannot be overlooked.

7. Toxicity - We are inundated with toxicity. Some of it, we can adapt to. Some of it, we cannot. Toxicity triggers a distinct chemical/hormonal response in the brain and sets off a chain of events throughout the entire body... inflammation being one of them. Look at the list about in the "stress" category - those are all sources of toxicity. To that list we can add environmental toxicity as well. Consider sources of toxicity from air, water, personal care products, household, garden, and lawn care products, cosmetics, heavy metals, vaccines, etc. It can be overwhelming to consider just how toxic our world has become. (It's why I believe that a regular cellular detoxification protocol is so important.)

8. Chronic Sleep Deprivation - Hopefully, you can see the connection here... deprivation (or deficiency) anywhere along the spectrum of 'things our body needs' can lead to a toxic, inflamed situation. However, even one night of

sleep deprivation (we're talking 4 - 5 hours of sleep here) has been shown to significantly raise the markers of inflammation!

9. Chronic Alcohol Consumption - Alcohol contributes to leaky gut, as well as bacterial and fungal/yeast overgrowth in the intestines. It's a highly concentrated dose of sugar, as well, triggering the body's insulin response.

10. Drug Use - Many prescription and over-the-counter drugs directly contribute to inflammation themselves. One of these is NSAIDS (non- steroidal anti-inflammatory drugs, like aspirin, ibuprofen, Celebrex, etc.). Research clearly indicates that even 3 days of taking over-the- counter drugs like ibuprofen can cause inflammation and a leaky gut. Another family drugs directly linked to gut inflammation is antibiotics. Antibiotics do not only attack the intended target bacteria - they wreak havoc on all bacteria, including the "healthy" bacteria throughout our intestinal systems that are so critical to our overall health and immune function.

11. Nutritional Deficiencies - As I made reference to earlier, deficiency means we're not getting what our cells require in order to achieve &/or

maintain a state of homeostatic cell function. This can lead to inflammation as a result of the lack of key 'ingredients' required for proper digestion.

12. Low Hydrochloric Acid in the Stomach - Most people think that indigestion and acid reflux are the result of having too much acid in the stomach. Actually, most of the time, it's just the opposite, especially as we get older. When we don't have enough HCL to break down our food properly, we can experience the burning sensation as particles of food that are not properly broken down stay in the upper digestive track for longer than they should (because the body is saying "hey, this food is too big for me to pass along to the small intestines!"). Or, if those food particles that are too large do get passed on to the small intestine, they cause breakdown of the intestinal lining, leading to leaky gut, which causes chronic inflammation.

(So, those acid pump inhibiting drugs you see on television? They end up causing the food to be pushed out of the stomach before it's efficiently broken down - so you stop feeling the burn - but now you've set the stage for much bigger problems with gut permeability, leaky gut,

inflammation, and setting the stage for an autoimmune

condition over time.)

1. Hormonal Imbalance - This is a big one! We're not just talking about reproductive hormones, or "women's" hormones, which many people still assume when you mention the word "hormonal"! Hormones are the chemical messengers for all the systems of our bodies and they play a critical role in every function. One example of the hormonal- inflammation connection is with the stress hormone, cortisol.

   When our adrenal system is fatigued from chronic stress or toxicity, we can burn through so much of our stress hormone supply that cortisol becomes depleted. Unfortunately, cortisol is one of the things that our body uses to control the inflammatory process, naturally!

   On the flip side, when there is inflammation, the hormonal receptors on the cell membrane end up not being so 'receptive' to the hormonal message attempting to be delivered. This clearly results in hormonal dysregulation - the message can't get to its intended destination, or the message gets skewed. A hormone drug or cream doesn't solve this dilemma.

2. Infections - Bacterial, viral, fungal, or parasitic. These chronic, often undetected and untreated,

infections cause inflammation as the immune system is relentlessly on the attack, trying to keep the infection under control. One of the simplest things we can do to offset potential infection, particularly in the gut, is to replenish the gut with healthy, immune empowering bacteria in the form of high-quality probiotics.

Severe Brain Trauma - Remember the critical connection between the gut and the brain? Here, it plays out in reverse. If there is brain injury, that, in turn, has been shown to cause leaky gut in as little as six hours or less! Of course, this leads to chronic inflammation over time if not properly addressed.

While this list can seem daunting and impossible to overcome, it's not. We can transition to a more "anti-inflammatory" lifestyle with relative ease.

Remember though, the "anti-inflammatory" approach will only get you so far. You've also got to heal & repair the gut, otherwise the inflammatory cycle can continue... even in response to "healthy" choices in diet, for example.

Please don't fret! It's not about being perfect. It's about making better choices, more often.

Stick to "real" food vs. synthetic factory foods & junk food, stay hydrated, move your body, add something like yoga to nurture your overall health, have an outlet for stress, get enough sleep, be grateful, remove as many sources of toxicity as you can... it's all good!

Every healthy choice adds up to make a positive difference and you'll never be able to take away a healthy choice that you made! Just focus of stringing more of them together each day, each week, for the long run. That's how health is created.

INFLAMMATION: TIPS TO HEAL YOUR SKIN AND BODY

Caring for your skin and maintaining its youth and luminosity, whether through quality skin care products or regular facials, may seem to many people a matter of vanity and indulgence. Let's be honest; to some degree it is. We want to look good, because when we look good we feel better about ourselves. But valuing your esthetic needs benefits you more than skin deep, especially when it comes to inflammation.

The skin is the largest organ in your body and it has a multitude of functions that are taken for granted. For example, not only is it the casing that wraps your musculature, skeletal structure and internal organs, it is like the bouncer in a nightclub. It makes sure only the right things get in, and keeps some of the most important ones from getting out. The skin also acts as a full-time garbage disposal by filtering waste, just like your kidneys, and its acidic pH makes it a hostile environment for bacteria to survive.

In the evolution of skin care there are many approaches to correcting aging concerns, including balancing hormones, protecting from UV radiation, correcting free-radical damage, and detoxification. Micro- injections have become more and more popular in recent years, aswell as sirtuin technology which focuses on activating the enzymes that prolong the life of cells. But what do you know about inflammation?

I'm guessing what comes to mind is probably swelling, redness, heat and perhaps even discomfort. If so, you're on the right track, butthat's not the inflammation I'm talking about. What's more, if you don't have rosacea, you're probably wondering what this has to do with you. What if I told you the inflammation I am referring to is an internal and silent inflammation that you neither see nor feel. To put it another way; it's not a matter of if you have inflammation, it's a matter of when you will see its effects and the actual toll it's taking on your skin (and body in general) over the years.

You see, there are two types of aging: Extrinsic and Intrinsic and I am pretty certain that what you've been treating up until now has only been

Extrinsic. Just as these names suggest, extrinsic aging happensoutside of the body and is influenced by all the factors you are already aware of: damaging radiation due to sun exposure, pollution, and other free- radical causing agents. By contrast, intrinsic aging occurs inside the body and its main governing factors are genetics and inflammation.

Inflammation is like stress. It has its benefits when it is the body functioning to protect itself. The fight or flight response and spike in adrenaline have been an important tool in the evolution of our species to ensure survival. However, chronically elevated levels of adrenaline - commonly known as stress- begins breaking down your immune system, making you more susceptible to illness.

By the same token, inflammation is the skin's response when an unknown element "attacks" the skin. Blood is rushed to the affected area (increasing heat and redness in the skin) to assist white blood cells in killing infection. Chronic inflammation (whether it's visible or not) keeps the skin in a heightened state of response. Every time this protective mechanism occurs, enzymes are released to destroy cells, including collagen and elastin, and free-radicals are released.

At this point you're most likely wondering what causes inflammation. As I've just mentioned, stress and diet are biggies, although stress seems to be the accepted norm in society today. And although, I'm not asking you to overhaul your current lifestyle, tweaking your diet AND using the appropriate skin care products will make a big, long-term difference not only in the beauty of your skin, but in your overall health.

Aging is not the only skin condition inflammation causes over time. Other common skin concerns include acne, pigmentation spots, sagginess, enlarged pores, dryness, dullness, reddening of the skin and flare-ups.

So how do you treat this inflammation? Too many times I've had clients that believe that the 'stronger' or harsher a product or treatment is, the better it must be. After all, it must mean it's more effective, right? Wrong.

Believe me, more aggressive treatments can be effective, and are at times necessary, depending on the condition of the skin and the results that need to be achieved. All peels, lasers and medical skin care treatments have their place. These treatments cause a wound response in the skin, which can have its benefits as long as you re-establish BALANCE and give your skin the tools it needs to properly heal and restore itself, maintaining its health from the inside-out.

Here are some basic steps to get you started on addressing

inflammation:

1. Begin supplementing your skin care with products that contain ingredients such as aloe, gingko biloba, allatoin, honey and chamomile. Skin growth factors (SGFs) are also key in healing and regenerating the skin.

2. Be sure to wear a broad-spectrum sunblock on a daily basis that contains titanium dioxide or zinc

oxide as active ingredients in a 6% or higher.

3. Avoid extremely hot water in washing your face or in your showers. Opt for lukewarm to cool water instead and even keep some skin care products in the refrigerator for that soothing, cooling effect.

4. Include fresh vegetables and fruits in your diet, along with whole grains and salmon. If you're not big on fish, Omega 3 and 6 fatty acid supplements are also effective at targeting the inflammation.

5. Avoid sugar and coffee as much as you can. Black and green tea are great caffeine alternatives, in addition to being full of antioxidants!

Having more beautiful, youthful and radiant skin doesn't necessarily mean completely altering your lifestyle, although it does call for some changes. Surgery, botox and fillers will eliminate wrinkles, but they don't change the quality and health of your skin. It's not about just a superficial quick fix if you're looking for long-term results, but rather a whole-listic approach that involves treating and healing the skin from

the inside-out. Who knows, you may even lose a few inches off your waistline!

Made in the USA
Middletown, DE
23 February 2021